THINK Yourself THIN

NATHALIE PLAMONDON-THOMAS

THINK Yourself THIN

The DNA System
to Reprogram Your Own Brain
to Lose Weight and Keep it Off

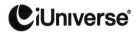

THINK YOURSELF THIN
THE DNA SYSTEM TO REPROGRAM YOUR OWN
BRAIN TO LOSE WEIGHT AND KEEP IT OFF

iUniverse books may be ordered through booksellers or by contacting:

iUniverse
1663 Liberty Drive
Bloomington, IN 47403
www.iuniverse.com
1-800-Authors (1-800-288-4677)

Because of the dynamic nature of the Internet, any web addresses or links contained in this book may have changed since publication and may no longer be valid. The views expressed in this work are solely those of the author and do not necessarily reflect the views of the publisher, and the publisher hereby disclaims any responsibility for them.

Any people depicted in stock imagery provided by Thinkstock are models, and such images are being used for illustrative purposes only.
Certain stock imagery © Thinkstock.

ISBN: 978-1-4917-8467-9 (sc)
ISBN: 978-1-4917-8468-6 (e)

Library of Congress Control Number: 2016900428

Print information available on the last page.

iUniverse rev. date: 1/18/2016

Disclaimer from Nathalie Plamondon-Thomas: While many of my clients have seen great results following this system, I cannot guarantee that it will work for you as results are different for everyone.

To contact Nathalie: www.dnalifecoaching.com

CONTENTS

1 A Sad Reality   **1**

2 Book Overview   **3**

3 How Did I Come to the Conclusion That the Brain Was Connected to Weight Loss?   **9**

4 What's in It for You?   **13**

    The logical mind   15

    The unconscious mind   17

5 What Didn't Work?   **23**

    Focus on Food   23

    There is no failure, there's only feedback.   23

    4 Stages of Learning   25

    Unconscious competence vs Self-Sabotage   28

    Habituation   29

6 What Did Not Work? Focus on Exercise   **34**

    Overweight Problem in Canada   34

    Plateau: Psychology or Physiology?   37

    Pressure vs Stress   38

7 The D.N.A. System   **41**

    Discipline   42

8 "D" for Desire   **44**

    Desire vs Want   44

9 Demand   **46**

10 Do Not...   **48**

11	Do It with Your Body and the Mind Will Follow	**52**
12	Dedicate	**56**
	Divide	57
13	Determine	**62**
	Determine the intention behind the desire of losing weight	62
	Determine your expectation with this book	65
14	Dare	**72**
15	"N" for New You	**86**
16	Neuro-linguistic Programming	**87**
17	Need	**89**
	People have all the resources they need to succeed.	89
18	Norm	**91**
	Each person has his or her own unique model of reality	91
19	Neurological Levels	**96**
20	Negative to Positive	**108**
21	Neuro Pathways	**119**
22	Negative Neuro Pathways	**126**
23	Nemesis	**129**
24	New You Activity	**134**
25	Neutralize the Past	**139**
26	"A" for Actualize	**143**
27	Amplify Positive Feelings	**145**
28	Anchoring	**148**
	Spacial Anchoring	151
29	Act and Merge	**153**
30	Am I Fixed for Good Now?	**157**
31	Aware	**159**
	Are you CHOOSING your life?	159

32 Anticipate   **161**

33 Alternate Behaviour   **167**

34 Accountable   **171**

35 Authentic   **173**

36 Adopt the Toothpaste Philosophy   **177**

37 Appreciate   **180**

38 About the Author - Who Is Nathalie Plamondon-Thomas?   **183**

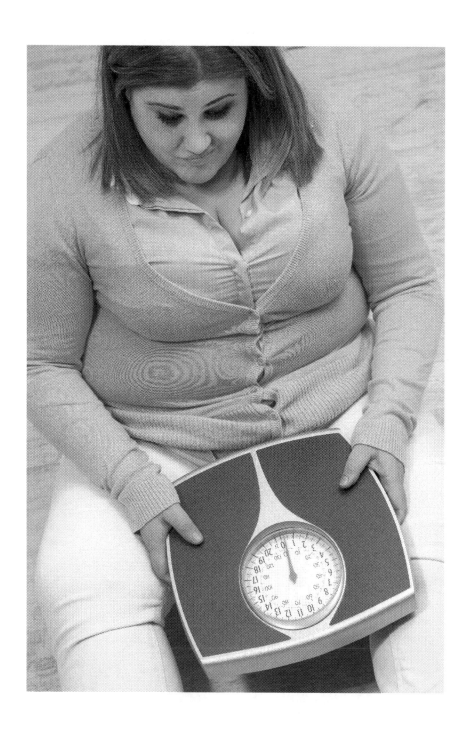

CHAPTER 1

A SAD REALITY

She was sound asleep, dreaming of a big outdoor venue with hundreds of guests. She was standing in her two-sizes-too-small satin dress and heels, close to the long buffet table filled with all her favourite delicacies on it. She was hardly paying attention to the guests around her, which seemed to be having a great time chatting and laughing. She was only pretending to follow their stories and would laugh when the others would laugh. In her head, her full attention was on the next thing she would take from the buffet table. She could not steer her attention away from the creamy cheeses, deep-fried appetizers, sausage rolls, nachos with seven-layer-dip, pastries, cupcakes and pies. Each bite was making her more and more excited and each bite was taking her further and further away from the conversations until she fully retracted from the mini group where she stood to go refill her plate for the fourth time. Her dress was becoming even more uncomfortable and she kept repeating in her head how much she hated being fat but yet, she kept shoving food into her mouth.

The alarm clock went off. For a moment she laid in bed wondering what the dream was all about... it was actually pretty close to her reality. Food occupied a big part of her life and she had never been comfortable in her skin, apart from the few periods of her life she spent at the "thin" phase of the 'yo-yo dieting' roller coaster she had been on for most of her adult life. She was 37, and fat. Period. Nothing worked and if for a short time some diets did work, it would

1

not be long before she would go back to her normal weight, which in her mind, was set to 'fat'.

Whenever a new diet would come on the market, she would put herself on it, fully motivated and cranked up. With great intentions she repeatedly told herself she did not want to be fat anymore and would follow with diligence whatever step, cure, detox, recipe, journaling, etc. required by the new fad. It would work for a while, then plateau, and then she would gain back the lost pounds with interest.

She never really liked what she saw in the mirror. She was barely able to handle the nasty negative self-talk that she would submit herself to whenever she glanced at the mirror coming out of the shower. She would just rather quickly wrap herself in the longest, biggest towel and robe she could find and stop looking at the mirror altogether.

She hated exercising as it was really hard and painful. She had signed up many times for memberships at different gyms and classes in her town and even though she was repeating in her head the 'no-pain-no-gain' slogan she had heard millions of times, she did not seem to feel motivated to become consistent with her training. She hated it and kept telling herself that it was hard and painful but that is what she had to do in order to stop being fat.

Every evening, she found comfort in her television shows. They were a big part of her life and would bring her into a different world. Somehow, the characters were her friends and much more consistent and less judgmental than her real friends who kept making her feel bad as she seemed to be treating herself every time they would go out. She would order the burger and fries or the deep fried calamari while her friends all seemed to pretend to actually like the salads that they would order. She preferred to order real restaurant food (not a darn salad) and her usual bottomless soda pop.

CHAPTER 2

BOOK OVERVIEW

You may or may not be able to relate to any of the behaviours in the above story. You too may feel that exercise is hard and eating healthy is boring. You may feel that it is easy to lose weight and yet have engrained an unconscious belief that no matter how motivated, you will always gain it back, with interest. This book is about teaching you how to change these limiting beliefs about yourself and about weight loss and how to program your brain to reach the weight you want and keep it off.

Can your brain really have anything to do with how you look and feel? It is no secret that the mind and the body are connected. The brain, being one of the most complex structures in the universe, has been the subject of studies and research for years.

This book is for you if:

- you feel that you are always on a diet
- you wonder what's wrong with you
- you hate looking in the mirror
- you have a hard time finding clothes that fit
- you have heard yourself say: "I eat my emotions"
- you have lost weight only to gain it back, with interest
- you think that losing weight is hard
- you think that food has control over you
- you can't seem to fit exercise in your schedule and when you do, it's a burden and you hate it.

DNA

In this book, you will learn about the D.N.A. System that I use with my clients. I have combined my experience of fitness, nutrition, Life Coaching and Neuro Linguistic Programming into a system that will show you how to reprogram your brain to lose weight effortlessly – and how to keep that weight off for good. I will share many examples with you about how my clients are being and have been successful in changing their life from the inside out. It is more a book about 'working in' vs. 'working out.'

In this book, we will review the two well-known components of weight loss: nutrition and exercise, in a way that will help you see the concepts differently, in a more mindful way. You will discover why your previous attempts to weight loss with nutrition and exercise may not have been as successful as you would have liked. I will introduce the D.N.A. system that I have been using with my clients. In your DNA are the fundamental and distinctive characteristics that qualify who you are. My most profound belief is that everybody has everything they need inside themselves. It is in your DNA. Somewhere inside, you know exactly what to do in order to be your best. I believe everybody is extraordinary and unique. Everyone can achieve the life that they desire. The know-how is all within them, waiting to be discovered.

I have been using these techniques and processes with my clients, which always followed a similar pattern. The first step was to teach them how the brain works and discover what they wanted, then we had to do some clean up, and finally we could install the new desires. As I was writing this book, I realized that I could regroup the information I wanted to present into three large categories. You will discover the complexity and power of the brain and how to elicit what you want (desire). You will learn how to make room for what you want and some techniques to clear any negative impact from your past (new you). And finally, you will learn how to program your brain with what you want (actualize).

The D.N.A. system stands for: DESIRE - NEW YOU - ACTUALIZE.

DESIRE

In the DESIRE part, you will learn how your mind has been conditioned for years to hate exercise and healthy food and how discipline starts in your head, with what you are programmed to love or hate. You will learn that you can demand what you want from your brain and it will execute your command. You will realize how your brain will always make you right. If you focus on being fat, your brain will make sure to stay this way. You will read how the "do not" and the "don't" in your language have contributed to how your brain is presently wired. You will understand that the brain is at the base of your actions as the mind and body are connected. I will show you a powerful demonstration of the placebo effect so you can see for yourself how you get whatever you expect. You will understand another reason why your old diets did not work was because they were temporary, as opposed to be built-in, like a definitive new habit.

You will learn how to find out what you really want by dedicating your efforts to one thing at a time, dividing your life into different segments (not just work and family) and determining what influences your weight loss.

Finally, this section will invite you to dare. Eliciting exactly what you want, aiming to have lots of choices and opportunities, and following your real intent behind your desires.

NEW YOU

In the NEW YOU section, you will be introduced to neuro linguistic programming, the science to reprogram your brain, from which I learned most of the principles and processes you will learn in this book. All this time you were looking for outside solutions - diets online, in books, with weight-loss products - while all you had to do was to look inside. The capabilities are within you waiting to be discovered. You have everything you need.

You will find out how your own model of reality has been formed and how you create your norms. Sometimes, we imagine constraints and barriers that do not exist. They may just be in our head. You will be amazed to discover how the brain has a specific way of organizing your thoughts following its neurological levels: environment, behaviour, skills, values and beliefs, identity and life purpose.

The NEW YOU section is also the clean up section. Not only you will discover how your model of reality was formed, you will also learn how to turn the negative into positive, how neuro pathways are formed and how to change your nemesis into a new you by neutralizing the past.

Once you've cleaned your old negative emotions and limiting beliefs, you will get to the ACTUALIZE part of the book where you will actually learn how to install the new desires you came up with in the first section. Techniques of anchoring, alternating behaviours, assuming excellence and acting will guide you into programming the NEW YOU.

ACTUALIZE

The ACTUALIZE section will also make sure you are aware of the choices you will continue to make once the new desires are installed and prepare you for an alternative in case some days, you face unexpected situations. You will learn how to become accountable to yourself and feel authentic by feeding your brain daily.

You will get a chance to practice the concepts right away in the book. I have included some brain exercises and techniques to start reprogramming your brain right away. I have adapted some techniques that I successfully use with my clients into simple processes that you will be able to use on your own. The exercises are there to help you start thinking yourself thin right away, as you read the book. You will be amazed at the results you get just by applying what you will discover in this book. Take the time to use the exercises and do them with care and time. After all, I suspect that this may not be the first book or tool you've purchased in order to lose weight. By making a commitment and applying yourself to take the time to really embrace these exercises and this new way of thinking, this book will be the last one you buy on the subject!

If you prefer to write your answers separately, you can download my free Think Yourself Thin workbook at <u>www.dnalifecoaching.com</u>.

You will notice lots of examples and sometimes repetition with the exercises. Change doesn't happen at a conscious level. Your logical mind (which I will explain further later on) is quite limited. Most of the processes you used before were based on your logical mind. However, change occurs at an unconscious level. You will discover how to get in touch with the most powerful portion of your brain: your unconscious mind. You know that we only barely touch the surface of the capabilities and potential of our brain. There is so much more we can tap into. Your unconscious mind will understand what I am talking about in the next chapters and will embrace these concepts. Your unconscious mind loves repetition, just like a child that wants to watch the same movie over and over. Your logical mind might think: ".... really? that same question again? I answered that already. It is kind of the same question. Wasn't this concept covered already?" Well, while your logical mind is busy trying to think that way, your unconscious mind is saying: "Yay! I love this stuff, can I hear it again one more time please?"

All this time you have been searching for a way to lose weight. You were reading techniques in books, magazines, web-resources, diets, gym memberships, and all you had to do was to look inside of you. Everything is there. All the tools you need. Search no more. Get ready to make your next trip to thin-land a one-way ticket to an enjoyable journey!

Before I get into the specifics of when and how we can use our brain to reach our weight loss goals, let me introduce myself and how I came to the conclusion, after years of practice with my clients, that weight loss can be achieved with other tools than a treadmill and some raw veggie sticks.

CHAPTER 3

HOW DID I COME TO THE CONCLUSION THAT THE BRAIN WAS CONNECTED TO WEIGHT LOSS?

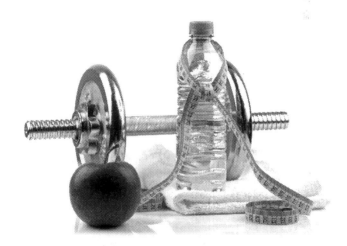

I am an award winning fitness professional and an NLP Master Practitioner and Life Coach. I have been teaching fitness class for over 28 years. It is a big part of my life. I am also a personal trainer and a nutrition and wellness specialist. In 2011, I wrote the book "When You're Hungry, You Gotta Eat" which continues to be the basis for numerous seminars and workshops.

Over the years of teaching and coaching, people have come to me for questions and guidance about weight loss. They all want the same thing. Stop being fat. They ask me for advice on exercise and on nutrition, they want to know the latest trend, the new bootcamp, the new superfood, the latest smoothie or recipe. They usually hire me to make them a nutrition program or an exercise plan.

It took me a few years to realize it, but I started to observe the reason why my clients were successful and realized that it had nothing to do with the exercise program I had given them, nor the menu they were following. The reason why they succeeded was because of their new way of seeing themselves. I realized that I was contagious as to the way I had been thinking myself and that I could transmit that knowledge and change their vision of themselves by changing their thoughts. The way I was brought up wired my brain a certain way and I never ever noticed that it was somehow unusual. I thought everybody was wired the same. I thought that it was normal to like healthy food and to enjoy exercise. Most people would tell me, well, that is easy for you, but for most people, it is hard and painful. So why was that? Why is that easy for me (and a select few) while the majority fails at it?

I started to dig more into it and observe my thoughts, ask more questions of my clients, started to be more specific as to digging into their internal dialogue and what words they were using to refer to themselves. What were they thinking about when they looked at themselves? How were they perceiving exercise and healthy food?

It has never been about the actual way to perform a bicep curl or the specific menu or superfood that I would put my clients under. All of that time, it was right in front of me. The reason why my clients were successful was because they were starting to think like me. I started to observe my friends around me, my co-workers, my participants, looking at who was thin, and who was struggling with their weight. What were they saying and thinking of themselves? What was their reality? What was their reset point that their body would always return to as they were programmed and conditioned to stay this way, no matter how successful the latest diet had been?

I realized that there was a constant in a lot of female clients. It often started with them wanting to lose weight with behaviours like eating and exercising. The successful ones would be the ones that changed their values and beliefs, not their behaviours. So I decided to use all the knowledge from what I studied in Coaching and in Neuro Linguistic Programming along with my personal and professional experience and those of my clients, to put together the D.N.A. system that will include an explanation on how the brain works and practical activities and techniques that were proven to work with my clients through my years of practice.

Although I still offer nutrition consultation and personal training along with teaching my fitness classes, I know now that unless the mind set is changed, there will not be any substantial and lifelong results. When a client wants to lose weight and asks me to give them nutrition advice, I simply smile and tell them: "You don't really need me to tell you what to eat, nor do you need me tell you how to exercise, there are millions of tips and strategies online and with your experience dieting all your life, you probably know more recipes than I do. What I can teach you is **how to feed your brain**."

When you read the *About the Author* section at the end of the book, you will realize that I drank the potion at a very young age and this comes naturally for me. The good news is that you will learn in this book that it doesn't even matter what kind of background or childhood you had. All mental states and skills are teachable and learnable. You will learn about Neuro Linguistic Programming which is the study of human excellence, the science of modelling great behaviours, using specific linguistic markers that your deeper self will understand and apply. You will be amazed at how easy and effortless it is to reprogram your own brain so that you can also benefit from this amazing way of thinking. Can you imagine how great your life will be when you can control your thoughts? When you can program your brain to do whatever it is you want to accomplish and, keeping in the subject of the present book, program yourself to be thin?

KEY CONCEPTS:

Desire to lose weight

+

Exercise

+

Nutrition

=

NOT ENOUGH!!!

Change in mind set

=

SUCCESS

CHAPTER 4

WHAT'S IN IT FOR YOU?

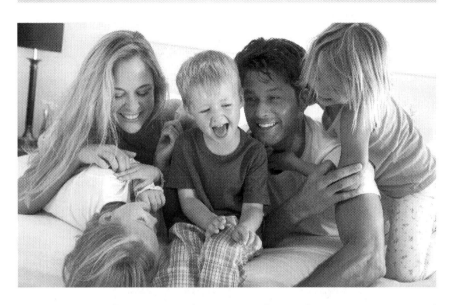

Most of us see our lives going by without noticing it and we wake up one day and 10 years of our life have gone by and we say: "I wish I had done this, or done that". What is on the back burner? What are the dreams and hopes that we put aside? With my clients, the first thing we do in a session is to assess what the client really wants. We answer the million-dollar question: "If you could do anything and be anything you want, what would it be?" Then we figure out ways to achieve it. Our mind is very complex but yet, it is quite simple. Whatever we dream, we can achieve. No mind will plant a seed unless it is able to grow the end-result. So whatever your dream is, it is possible. Otherwise your mind would not let you even dream it.

I have a client who wanted to get pregnant. She had a child already so she knew that biologically it was possible for her and her husband to have children. They had been trying for a year but it wasn't working. We did a few sessions together and we determined that she was focusing on the wrong thing: "not being able to get pregnant" and was stuck; she was not able to define her positive outcome clearly. We re-defined what she wanted moving forward instead of focusing on what had not worked. Since discovering how her new mind set could help her in giving birth to her second baby, she has been using this new way of thinking in everything she does. She now lives a very busy and fulfilled life with her husband and their three children (yes they even had a third).

There are different reasons why people hire a coach. I coached a woman in Ontario who wanted to find a boyfriend. She actually found someone shortly after which she spend a few months with, giving her the self-confidence she needed in order to be her best and then met Mr Right and really fell in love. They are now married and travel the world together. I had a client who wanted to quit smoking. He has now since signed up for his first half-marathon and never felt better. I helped a businessman who wanted to advance his career. As it turned out, he realized that spending time with his family was more important to him than the promotion he had been applying for. I coached a woman in Saudi Arabia (I coach people worldwide either by phone or over Skype) who wanted to change her work place and she is now pursuing her vision in a non-profit organization in Germany. I coached a female police officer who wanted to lose weight; she knew how to exercise and ate well but was stuck with the last 15 pounds. She was stuck in her work and it reflected in her weight. She went for training and got extra skills that moved her to the next level on the ladder and she is now back to her desired weight. She loves her job and especially how her uniform fits now.

Most of the time my clients know the answers to their problems; it's inside their brain but their brain is not revealing the solution to them. Things happen and we respond to them. A problem is something that would not be a problem if we knew how to respond to it. We have to dig in our unconscious in order to find the solution. If we knew the solution right away, it would not be a problem.

I use the D.N.A. system to help people figure out what they want. I will elaborate more on the system later. For now, let's just say that I help them connect with their unconscious mind by clearing what is in the way, with specific processes, and I ask powerful questions in order for their brain to reveal the pathway. It becomes clear to them; they know what they want and they know what to do.

The specific processes are used to reprogram my clients' brains into becoming whatever they want to be. Some clients are just tired of feeling that they can do better and be better, some have decisions to make and are torn apart between two choices, some want to make changes to their life, some are just sometimes wishing they were more *like this* or *like that.* I teach them that they can be whatever they want to be.

Your brain is the most complex structure of the Universe. Asleep or awake it controls every moment, every movement and every thought of your Life. Think about it: Do you have to tell yourself to breathe? To swallow? To blink? Your brain controls it all without you having to think about it.

THE LOGICAL MIND

We use our logical mind in the surface in our day-to-day. Your logical mind is the voice you hear in your head all the time. The one you use to make decisions. We actually give our logical mind lots of responsibilities and place lots of hope as to the extent of its power. The logical mind can process an average of between five and nine pieces of information at the same time. So while you are reading this book, you are more likely also able to notice an average of seven other things. For example, as you read, you can picture yourself understanding these concepts, you can see yourself in the new outfit you will buy when you reach your desired weight, you can see what lays on your desk, hear if there is music playing in the background, notice that your pants feel uncomfortable, (and unfortunately depending on your actual programming and the way you think at this time), tell yourself that this book sounds too good to be true and that it will probably be another one of your unsuccessful multiple attempts to lose weight. You can do all of these things at the same time. Does it sound great? Your logical mind looks really powerful right? Just wait until you hear about the best part of your brain.

According to the research of Dr Raj Rahunathan Ph.D. we generate between 12,000 and 50,000 thoughts per day. Unfortunately, up to 70% of these thoughts are negative. We wonder what is wrong with us? Why is everybody else thin except us? We question why we haven't been chosen and tell ourselves we are probably not good enough. We think we would have time to exercise if we didn't have to take care of everyone else. We think everyone is better and knows more than us. These negative thoughts, either looking for approval or control, or demonstrating feelings of inferiority, represent most our daily internal dialogue. Sadly.

When you start paying attention to everything you tell yourself, you realize why your efforts for weight loss have been in vain. Would you want to be your friend if you talked to them the same way you talk to yourself?

Now our logical might not be that great after all right? And all these years, we solely relied on it for the most important decisions in our life.

Now the good news is that the voices inside your head have volume controls. You can make them louder, you can make them softer, you can make them say what you want to hear and in whatever tone of voice. We will learn all of this in the NEW YOU and ACTUALIZE sections of this book. For now, let's have a look at another part of your mind.

THE UNCONSCIOUS MIND

While the logical mind is busy talking down to you, the unconscious mind is busy working, understanding everything, down in the deep structure of our self. The unconscious mind can handle over two million pieces of information every second. (While our little logical mind was only able to hand seven on average). Everything you have seen, done, thought, heard, felt is organized in your deeper structure waiting for your recall. Your unconscious mind sees everything. It reads all the signs and advertising while you drive to work. It hears every conversation around you, whether you are paying attention or not. It feels all the non-verbal signs that others are communicating to you without their own knowledge. It captures all the "behind-the-scenes" details that the logical misses. It takes all the info, it deletes, distorts and filters everything to create your own model of reality.

Your unconscious mind has so much information for you. It is dying to tell you. The problem is that people are not trained to think with their unconscious mind. Before today, you might even have thought that the unconscious mind was a one-way drawer. You may have thought that the logical mind is the one we use for thinking and that the unconscious mind is the one we use for storing. Have you ever lost something that you had in your hand minutes before? You know you put it somewhere. You start thinking with your logical mind and wonder where you put it? Where can it be? You had it just now? Where did it go? The reason why you can't seem to find it is because you are asking the wrong part of your brain. Your logical mind was probably busy with six other things and did not notice what you did with it. You want to ask your unconscious mind. It knows. Always. After all, it was you that put it somewhere. You are not asking your unconscious mind to read somebody else's mind. Just yours.

Whatever we plant in our subconscious mind and nourish with repetition and emotion will one day become a reality.
Earl Nightingale

I could spend pages and pages giving you stories of my life as I am constantly using my unconscious mind to find things. One day, we were looking for the iPad. There are only two of us living in a small house. The iPad is always in the kitchen. My husband and I are both tidy people and there isn't any clutter that could have been piled up on top of it. We were both quite puzzled as to where it went. After a few minutes of searching, I said: "Well, I guess I will have to ask my unconscious mind where it is, I am sure it saw it somewhere if my husband put it there, or it remembers where I put it, if it was me." As I was thinking about my unconscious mind, the first thought that came to my mind was to give up the search and that the iPad would turn out eventually. Somehow, I got told by my unconscious mind to go back to work. That is what I did. I got back to my computer and printed a document that I needed to print and when I reached to the printer to grab my report, the iPad was sitting on the printer, right there. I smiled and thanked my unconscious mind. Anchoring the fact that it always knows.

At the airport, I was waiting at the gate to get on the plane. At time of boarding, I reached into my purse pocket for my boarding pass and my Nexus card. The boarding pass was there but my ID had disappeared. I started to panic. It was time to board. I know I had it to go through security so it could not be far. I started to frantically take everything out of my purse and my travel bag until I suddenly talked myself out of it. I stopped the search. I sat down and relaxed. I was there when I put the Nexus card somewhere. Why don't I ask myself? Why don't I question the real part of me that knows? As soon as I said that to myself, the first thought that came to my mind was to glance at my shiny boots. The shoe-shine-guy!!! I must have left the card when I got my boots polished. I ran back to the shoe-shine kiosk and as I approached, he smiled at me and reached in his shirt pocket to hand me my Nexus card. He said: "I knew you would be back for it!". I gave him a big tip and a hug and ran back to my gate to board the plane. Again, I took a second to thank my unconscious mind and anchor the fact that it works every time. Reinforcing the belief that I can easily access my deeper structure.

Using the D.N.A. System, my clients are able to make their logical mind and unconscious mind communicate together so that they have access to that deeper structure, where everything is clear and simple. The answers are all within them, waiting to be accessed. In the airport example, I could have let stress and panic get in the way. I sure did for a few seconds. It is not that I never go there. I just don't stay there long. With practice, you get used to exploiting the power of your unconscious. When the layers and layers of negative emotions and negative thoughts have been removed, there is a clear path between your logical and unconscious mind. This communication with our deeper structure is one of the most powerful techniques I teach my clients.

We also work together on their priorities and make sure that they advance their projects instead of leaving them on the back burner. We work on changing the attitude: *"if it happens, it happens"* into: *"it will happen because I will make it happen"*.

Most of my clients come to me because they are tired of feeling that they are not in charge of their destiny and tired of watching their life happening to them. They are tired of having tried lots of methods to reach their goals, only to get a temporary boost and then get back to the same old rut again.

I have a passion for people. I love listening to what people say. The power hidden in the words we use everyday is underrated. We will see in this book how we can use the power of words to serve our goals in life. I don't suggest nor do I advise my clients. I just ask the questions in order for them to generate the solution themselves. People need to make their own decisions in order to stick with the consequences. Their own brain needs to generate the idea. So I don't give advice. The solution sometimes comes to me very quickly in some cases. Other times, I am totally off track and my intuition is not at all what the outcome of the session turns out to be, which doesn't matter because the sessions are not about me but about my client. They are the ones who find their own answers. I can only ask powerful questions and help their subconscious mind deliver them the answer that will serve them best.

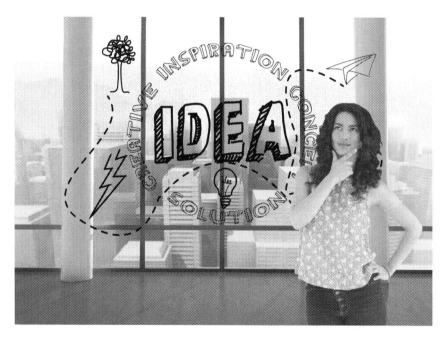

Have you ever told something to someone so many times and then 4 months later they have the brilliant idea of doing what you had been suggesting? You want to shake them and say: "Well, that is what I have been telling you to do for months!!!" But they were not listening. They have to be the ones getting the idea themselves. When you told them, at the time, their brain was not ready to process that information. Unless they generate the idea themselves, you can tell them all you want, but it isn't going to work.

Clients and friends often ask me for advice, or they want my opinion on something. My on-going response is always: "It doesn't matter what I think. It doesn't matter what anybody thinks. I was not there. I don't know all the details about this. I don't have your background, your experience nor your values. Why don't you ask someone that was there all your life; that noticed everything; that heard every conversation and even picked up on all the non-verbal information that nobody else picked up on? Ask your unconscious mind. It knows exactly what to do. The best moment to do so is at night before you go to sleep. When you get to bed tonight, intentionally ask your unconscious mind to recall every piece of information you have on the subject and give you a clear vision the next morning. It is important to ask your unconscious mind to do this WHILE YOU ARE PROFOUNDLY ASLEEP. (Otherwise, it could keep you up all night). You must specify that while your logical mind is recharging and getting long hours of rejuvenating sleep, you want your unconscious mind to work in the background and give you answers in the morning.

I often use that technique when I know I have a deadline to write an article or a specific task. I ask my unconscious mind to write it overnight so that when I wake up the morning after, the words come easily and effortlessly to me. I even use my unconscious mind to pack before a trip. It knows every single piece of clothing I own, it knows which ones I prefer, which ones are the most comfortable and appropriate for the trip that is ahead of me, some say that it can even tell the future and that it knows if it is going to be sunny or cold. So let your unconscious mind pack for you too. Usually, the morning after asking my unconscious to make the list for me, I only need 15 minutes and my suitcase is closed!

Imagine how great your life will be when you can access all the knowledge and the experience that your unconscious mind has for you!

We spend so much time dwelling on our problems that it becomes a habit to do so. We become good at having problems and if they go away, there is a sense of emptiness that we feel the need to fill with some other problems. Isn't that weird? In coaching, we spend time focusing on what we want instead. The actual problem doesn't really matter. We make it disappear to direct our energy into what we want. For some clients, it so happened that I never even knew why they hired me. The actual problem didn't matter. No need to dwell on it. It is all about moving forward. We only focused on the next step to get them closer to what they wanted, instead of using their time talking about what they did not want anymore.

Now you have a better understanding of my role as a life coach and what I am about to teach you. Even with the multitude of reasons why people hire me, the constant is always the same. They always have all the answers to their problems within themselves and you are about to learn how to access it.

KEY CONCEPTS:

The logical mind can only handle 5 to 9 things at a time while the unconscious mind can manage over 2 million pieces of information per second.

We tend to only ask input from our logical mind, which is negative 70% of the time.

People don't tend to implement other people's advice. They need to generate the solution themselves.

We should ask our unconscious mind for answers. They reside inside us in our deeper structure, which can be accessed once all the negative emotions have been cleared.

If you want advice, don't ask around. Ask yourself.

CHAPTER 5

WHAT DIDN'T WORK?

FOCUS ON FOOD

Every action that we do generates a result. Whether it is a successful result or not, every attempt at losing weight will generate a result. It may or may not work. Or it will work for a while and the weight might come back. Your own past experience is there to teach you what did not work so that you can try something else. If nothing changes, nothing changes. If you need to lose weight, if you want to look and feel better and you need help getting motivated, this book is exactly what you have been waiting for.

THERE IS NO FAILURE, THERE'S ONLY FEEDBACK.

If your weight loss plan didn't work, then you need to get feedback about why. Ask yourself what worked and what didn't work. Each action will give you a result. Success or not, whatever you do, you will obtain a result. Every action will give you information. This result will teach you a great deal about the action you did. Was it successful? Did it work? Did it last? What can you do differently now to generate a different result?

I like to think that everything I do is only a trial. An experiment. I believe that we all have a certain percentage of success that follows us around. What I mean by that is that we all do things and we get a success rate of let's say 20%. That means that 1 action out of 5 generates a good reaction. The other 4 things are guiding us there. Learning what doesn't work so that we can get to the magic 5th successful time. Every time we do something that doesn't work, that means that we get closer and closer to reach the one that will work. Each move in our life is a stepping-stone towards something else. Everybody we meet, every article or blog we read, every action we do, they are there temporarily to bring us to the next level. Living your life with this philosophy will help you react better to what you had seen in the past as failure. The next time something doesn't work out just say: "Alright! That means that I am now at or 3 out of 5 and I only have two or more things to learn before I get it right!"

I guess you are starting to know me by now. Do I need to mention here that I chose to believe that my success rate is 100%? I chose to believe that I am the luckiest person on earth and that I always succeed 100% of the time. I succeed at learning whatever I needed to learn with what I was aiming for. I succeed at growing. I succeed at getting better and improve myself. Then I have another goal: To do it again and learn some more.

Success does not consist in never making blunders, but in never making the same one a second time.

Josh Billings

Most people with weight issues have actually done a lot work with nutrition and food in their life. You have counted calories, you know how many points is worth everything you put in your mouth, you have a calories tracker, you filled out numerous food journals, tried all the diets and combinations possible, you cut dairy, gluten, fat, carbs, proteins, all at once or separately... How is that working for you?

I am not saying that food is not important in your weight loss journey. What you chose to put in your mouth is actually crucial. I cannot stress enough the important of eating a clean diet. What I am saying here is that I will not teach you what is healthy and what is not. I will not give you recipes. I will not tell you what is the next superfood. There is no shortage of information about the specific food to eat. You already know all of that. This book is not about what to eat and when to eat, nor what to avoid. Instead, I will teach you how to program your brain to reach for that healthy food naturally and effortlessly. The food section of this book is to make you think about food differently.

Let's talk about food now in a different and mindful way. The same way we do a lot of things without noticing that we are great at doing them, we want to start thinking about food in a way that will serve our goals.

4 STAGES OF LEARNING

This brings me to introduce the four stages of learning. All learnings and behavioural changes are unconscious.

Unconscious incompetence

At first, we don't know what we don't know. We think that being fit and eating healthy has to be hard. This is the stage of *unconscious incompetence*. I have great news for you. As you are reading this book, you have already stepped over that stage. This is the first day of the rest of your life. You can never go back to not knowing what you are about to find out. Your life will be changed forever! You will never be able to not know this anymore. You may have to work at applying all the techniques that I will show you, but you are not unconsciously incompetent anymore because you have been made conscious that these techniques exist.

Conscious incompetence

By being introduced to the idea that eating healthy can be easy, we now know that it is possible. We are not skilled yet but we know that it can be done. This is the stage of *conscious incompetence*. We start practicing and learning.

Conscious competence

Then it is *conscious competence*. Now we are good at it. We know what we are doing and our skills become habitual and consistent. We still have to consciously think about how to phrase our thoughts and how to apply the techniques that you have learned but they become very easy.

Unconscious competence

The last stage is reached when the skills become automatic. This is the ultimate goal. Once we are able to make choices without even noticing or thinking about it, we have reached the level of *unconscious competence*. Have you ever been on the wheel of your car and arrived at destination and thought to yourself: "Am I already here? How did I even get here? I was not even paying attention." You don't have to think anymore about what to do when you see a red light or a green light, you just drive and everything is automatic.

Every artist was first an amateur.

Ralph Waldo Emerson

The unconscious is where we can begin problem solving. Once we have done something for a while, we become unconsciously competent and get unconscious skills. The problem is that we can develop bad habits that way, become discouraged or depressed, thinking that dieting is hard, exercising is tough, etc.

There are lots of things in our lives that we do automatically. We never have to pay attention while brushing our teeth in the morning. We just do it. In the same way, we are able to avoid doing lots of things because of the way our brain is programmed.

Here is an example (for the record, this example doesn't apply if you are a man or if you are a man with a beard.) If you are a woman, is there a man in your house? My husband shaves every morning, and when I go into the bathroom in the morning and see his razor and shaving cream on the counter, I don't have to resist the temptation to shave my face. I'm a woman and I don't do that. It's something that's so clear in our heads that we don't even think of doing it. We resist it very easily.

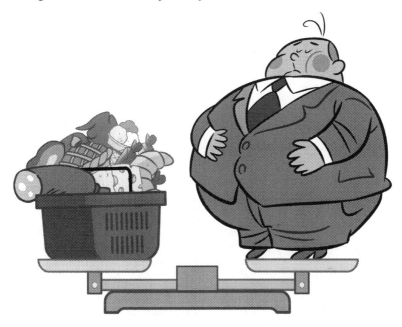

That's how we have to think when we encounter unhealthy foods. In the bakery section at the grocery store, do you buy a chocolate cake and strawberry cake and cheesecake and cookies and croissants? Are there some things you can go without and that you simply don't buy? Yes, you are capable of choosing and you do it all the time.

I had a client who always said, "I have no self-control." Yet, when she went grocery shopping, she actually did show self-control. She would beat herself up because she bought chips but she managed to resist the cookies, cakes and lots of other unhealthy things.

UNCONSCIOUS COMPETENCE VS SELF-SABOTAGE

How do we become unconsciously competent at choosing what to eat instead of giving in to the self-sabotage? Why is it that, for some specific foods, we think that they are stronger than us? We believe that some foods have power over us? It is just a question of programming. I hate the word downfall. I hear it so often. People keep programming themselves to be weak with some particular food. They say: "oh for me, salty stuff is my downfall", or "sweets are my downfall". So they are programming the brain that when in presence of these foods, to be weak and to succumb to the temptation.

In fact, we can only hold on to a state of mind for approximately 90 seconds. A craving doesn't really last long anyways before it goes away. It is not about resisting techniques. Everybody can resist for 90 seconds. Eating healthy doesn't have to be hard, and doesn't have to be about going against what you desire. It doesn't have to be boring either. It is about working at the source so that the desires change into healthy ones. It is going to become as easy as resisting shaving your face (if you are a woman). You are not a man, why should you shave? It is not a habit of yours. You don't buy EVERYTHING in the grocery store. There are some things that you don't buy. Easily. You just don't buy them. You don't need any "will power" to do so.

When you buy something you shouldn't, or order something you shouldn't at the restaurant, or grab something in your cupboard, or eat a 2nd serving, etc., who gives the call? Who is asking you to do so? Your brain is. What if your brain was conditioned to stay thin instead? Would it still give you the order of wanting this or that?

When you're eating something that you have programmed your brain to like, your brain tells you to go and get a second portion, so it seems that your brain is playing tricks on you. If you know that you don't need a second portion, and yet your brain tells you to go and get it, then something is wrong in your brain. Why are you working against yourself? Why are you self-sabotaging?

Why is your brain ordering you to grab that ice cream or that 2nd serving? It's because you are focusing on the wrong thing: Losing extra weight and stopping being fat. Your brain hears **Extra Weight** and **Being FAT.** We will learn how your brain works and how to succeed with the D.N.A. System in order to program it for being thin and staying healthy and fit, beautiful, adorable, desirable, and everything you wrote in the exercise above.

HABITUATION

Another way of talking about food from a 'brain' point of view is to mention the phenomenon of *habituation.* There is a study by Dr. Mehmet Oz about habituation.[1] It has to do with the brain and is related to portion controls or treats. There's an area in the brain where you receive the sensation when you eat the first bite. The first bite will give you five times the pleasure as your second bite. The pleasure decreases with each bite. If there were no habituation process, then you would keep eating and eating. Dr. Gary L. Wenk, Professor of Psychology and Neuroscience at The Ohio State University, demonstrates in his book *Your Brain on Food,* that a certain area of our brain controls the excitement about food. The pleasure given by the first bite decreases as we eat, until we don't even get any pleasure anymore. So we stop eating. Dr Wenk's research shows that if you visualize yourself eating before you actually eat you will decrease your portion size by 50%. Research also shows that you can get the same pleasure without even eating, just by visualization!

---

[1] http://www.doctoroz.com/article/your-imagination-can-make-you-thin

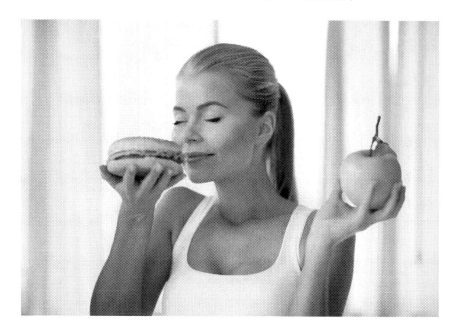

The good news is that you can recreate the pleasure just by thinking about it. You can get the same pleasure by visualizing eating the caramel-filled chocolate as actually eating it. Pretend, as it goes into your teeth and coats your teeth and the sides of your mouth and imagine it as it gets mushy and you have to clear your mouth with your tongue, and you really feel like you had that chocolate. Try it. It works!

We can use this theory to our advantage. The trick is to start habituation before we begin our meal. About half an hour before you start eating, visualize yourself eating the meal you will be having. If you do this, you will eat less because you'll feel fuller when you start.

My life changed when I actually discovered that, when faced with copious desserts, I could chose to only eat a few bites. There is no need to eat the whole dessert in order to get the satisfaction. You may have already mastered the technique of only eating a few bites and then pushing it aside. Imagine how you can now strengthen that technique by using the phenomenon of habituation. If you get given a piece of dessert at the office, or when invited at friend's house for dinner, take a moment to put it aside and just have it in your head first. When you're ready, just eat one real bite and then push it to the side and announce: "I'm full". Feel the pleasure of eating one bite, then stop. That is all you need.

Use the habituation method to strengthen your good eating habits. First, you might want to have a look at your diet and see if there is any change that needs to be addressed. You may need to include more plant-based products, drink more water, include more veggies or whatever your nutrition discoveries are teaching you. Theses changes alone will help you a great deal in your weight loss goals. The problem comes when you have changed your whole food pantry and still don't seem to be losing the weight that you want. You eat lots of salads, you make your own salad dressing with first-cold-pressed virgin oils, you don't use refined flour or sugar anymore, you don't buy any packaged goods, you replaced your pasta with zucchini, you only eat lean meat and lots of plant based proteins, and on an on. Why are you still not fitting in your skinny jeans? You might want to address portion control. Once we get used to healthy food and we start loving it, it can get easy to eat too much of it. That is when habituation comes handy. Have you ever heard yourself say: "I don't understand, I eat clean, I eat well and I can't seem to be able to get rid of the last ten pounds".

With this new method, you can think about the salad that you have packed for lunch ten minutes before eating it. If you eat out, you might want to stick to a few things that you know are healthy and re-order the same things, so that you can *habituate* while you wait for the server to bring your food. When you receive your meal, you will already have started the process in your head. Eating things that you know will help in the sense that not only you know that they are healthy for you, and also, you know what they taste like. A new flavour on your palate might trigger for you to eat more of it because it is new to you. That's another reason to eat at home or pack a lunch as often as possible. It's easier to *habituate* with foods that you're familiar with. Do I have to mention here that you might want to stay away from the all-you-can-eat buffets? Again, this is not a nutrition book. I will leave this one up to you to figure out.

The senses are also a great way to get satisfaction when it comes to cravings. It doesn't have to be the taste of the food that satisfies your craving. It can be the smell. Test it: order a salad and smell the fries from the neighbour's table and get the same pleasure!

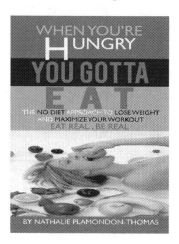

If you want more detailed information on nutrition (if you think you are not yet at the stage that you feel confident in your knowledge about nutrition,) pick up a copy of my book _When You're Hungry, You Gotta Eat_ on Amazon.com or get it for free by registering to my newsletter on www.dnalifecoaching.com. You can refer to this book for more detailed info about food and exercise. I explain in layman's terms how your brain processes information about hunger and satiety and how you can use that knowledge to lose weight. I teach you to focus on what you CAN eat (the "No-Diet" Approach).

I also give you tricks and tips on the myths and the facts about the trends, calculations on how to find your optimal weight and find out how many calories you should be eating every day, how to read labels, what to eat when you train, before & after your workout as well as some common sense information that you might already know but on which I will motivate you to put in practice. It is a no-diet approach to lose weight and maximize your workout.

KEY CONCEPTS:

There is no failure, only feedback

The four stages of learning

Unconscious Incompetence - You don't know you are not good at it, you don't know "it" exists
Conscious Incompetence - You know you are not good at it
Conscious Competence - You are good at it and you have to focus and think about it
Unconscious Competence - You are good at it and do it with your eyes closed, easily, effortlessly

Unconscious competency vs. self-sabotage

The way you think about food and your beliefs around your eating habits are causing you to self-sabotage your efforts to reach your weight-loss goals. YOU give the call.

Habituation

Thinking about food and rehearsing the eating process beforehand can help you with portion control. You can still enjoy less of it and yet, get the same mental satisfaction.

CHAPTER 6

WHAT DID NOT WORK? FOCUS ON EXERCISE

OVERWEIGHT PROBLEM IN CANADA

Statistics Canada is showing that, in 2014, 54% of Canadians were overweight or obese. That means more than one in two people are overweight. Think about it. There are two people in a room. Let's say you and a friend. One of you is overweight. Ouch. This is true for 61.8% of men and 46.2% of women.[2] This is scary because when you're overweight, it not only affects your quality of life and your self-confidence, it is also dangerous to accumulate fat around your organs. Obesity is not only a 'visual' problem; it can degenerate into all kinds of diseases and health issues. Consequently, at some point in their lives, over 60% of Canadians are dieting.

A lot of people join the gym and they only go a few times. That's the problem that we will talk about in this book: the fact that people don't stick with their intentions. Four out of ten overweight people spend money trying to slim down. Most people go for the quick-fix method. One quarter ask for help from doctors or dieticians, but three-quarters of people do it alone. The biggest challenge is to keep the weight off and it's very hard to do without support. If there's no support, 90% will regain the weight. 23% of Canadian teenagers weigh more than they should and are considered obese. This has

---

[2] Government of Canada - Statistics Canada - http://www.statcan.gc.ca/tables-tableaux/sum-som/l01/cst01/health82b-eng.htm.

more than doubled since 1985 since the arrival of video games and Internet and other technology. 40-60% of these teenagers will remain obese into their adult lives.

These facts are simply about the overweight problem. I could go on an on with statistics about degenerative diseases that are influenced or caused by the fact that our population is overweight. New diagnostics are growing every year for High Blood Pressure (5.3 million Canadians - 17% of the population), Asthma (2.5 million - 8%), Diabetes (2 million\ - 6.7%).[3]

Can you imagine what losing weight can do for these millions of people affected by any of the above? I am not talking about self-image here. I am talking about getting off your pills. How great will that feel when you can reverse the effect of your condition by introducing exercise into your life, easily and unconsciously? When it becomes naturally part of your life, just like brushing your teeth.

Again, this book is not about the benefits of exercising, nor how to perform a bicep curl or a squat. This book is about your brain and how to use it to get to exercise. Exercise doesn't have to be hard. It doesn't have to be boring. You are going to start feeling empowered and will become fitter, stronger and way more flexible than you ever imagined you could be. You don't need to worry about how you're going to feel and whether you're going to end up out of breath every time you do something because as you lose the weight, trust me, it's going to get easier and easier.

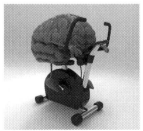 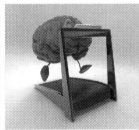 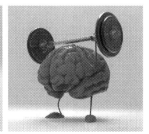

---

[3] Government of Canada - Statistics Canada - http://www.statcan.gc.ca/tables-tableaux/sum-som/l01/ind01/l3_2966_1887-eng.htm?hili_health49)

There's always going to be one type of exercise that you like. Maybe it's yoga, or swimming, or walking. Whatever it is, exercise empowers you. It has only good benefits, but it's just a matter of finding the one you like, and then you'll go back. Find the one thing that makes you feel like it's "me" time when you do it, and you'll love it. And if you don't love it, tell yourself that you do love it, fake it until you become it.

Put on comfortable clothes and running shoes and walk briskly away from your house for 15 minutes, then turn around and walk back home. You just went on a 30 minute walk!

What if you had more energy to enjoy your family and your family could enjoy you and you could live longer to be with them? Exercise has to be part of your life. It is a natural part of all healthy people's lives. When you're fit you don't have to worry about anything—you can walk for as long as you want, you don't get all sweaty just carrying the groceries, you can run after the bus if you are late without having to shower when you get to work nor be sore for two days. When you go shopping, you buy clothes and they fit right away! You don't have to worry about forgetting something upstairs, you just run up and back without any problem.

When exercise is part of your life, you live longer, healthier with a better mind-set, less stress, more self-confidence and life is good. You are also less at risk of developing serious health problems such as diabetes, heart disease, and stroke.

You are able to get the most out of life and you have enough energy to enjoy your family again and they enjoy the NEW YOU! Imagine the same you in a healthier and slimmer version. When you exercise, not only you feel better, you feel better about yourself. Exercising should be at the top of your priority list. We all agree with all the benefits of exercise. However, this book is more about working "in" than working out.

PLATEAU: PSYCHOLOGY OR PHYSIOLOGY?

As we are covering the subject of exercise, this is the perfect place to address this question that I get all the time from my clients and participants. • *I can lose weight, but then I get to a plateau. Why does that happen all the time?*

When a person weighs 200 lbs., they expend energy while walking to lift 200 lbs. However, once they lose for example 20 lbs., now they only have to lift 180 lbs. while walking and therefore not as much energy is expended, so not as many calories are required. With every ten pounds of weight lost, a re-evaluation needs to be carried out. Let's say you start an exercise routine and you are consistent at it for a month. You went from no exercise to hitting the gym three times per week. You had a personal trainer at first that got a program designed for you and this routine gave you great results for the first month. You were happy because, knowing that muscle weighs more than fat (hence the reason why we should not rely on the scale in order to decide whether or not our efforts are productive), you were seeing your body composition change and felt stronger and more toned. Then, during the second month, the results stopped being noticeable. You started thinking that exercise worked a bit at the beginning but it not really worth it anymore. You gave up and the rest is history.

What actually happened is that you had reached a plateau. It is necessary to always re-evaluate our level of fitness as we progress and avoid getting into the habit, or the comfortable zone, that slows down our results. As we get stronger, we can do more, we can do better, we can run faster, we can exercise harder and get to the next level. Once something becomes easy, we tend to pat ourselves on the back and think that we have succeeded and that it is over. We assume that we have reached the top level of fitness. Well, guess what? I am sorry to be the one to break the news to you, but there is always another level. Being comfortable and working out at only 30% of your maximum effort is not going to get you out of your plateau! You have been working hard to get to 180lbs from your 200lbs and it is important to celebrate that success. You rock! But your brain sees that success as the end of the task that it was assigned to achieve. Not only you need to re-evaluate your workout routine, (run faster, or longer, lift heavier weight, jump higher in your Zumba class), you also have to reprogram yourself to whatever is the next level that you want to reach. Once programmed, your brain will do the rest. You are now a size 8, that is what you dreamed of. But you still think you would like to get to the next size down. So you need to program yourself and convince yourself that you are a size 6.

Let's move on into the book so that we can learn how to get the proper mind set that will take us to the next level.

PRESSURE VS STRESS

What is the difference between pressure and stress?

Pressure is external. It is what happens to us in our lives. It is surrounding us every day. It is your alarm clock not going off, it is traffic, it is running out of milk, it is your boss holding you accountable for extra work, it is your child that is not feeling well, it is an unexpected expense, it is one of your parents falling ill etc. So all that external pressure is presented to you every day and it is affecting you.

This external pressure creates stress in your body. (Unless you are adopting the toothpaste philosophy that we will see later on in the book.) So stress is internal. A good way to get rid of stress is to take some time for yourself and focus, meditate or have a good sweat! Any type of exercise will help you get rid of the stress, momentarily. Yes, the external pressure will still be there, but it will not affect you anymore, for the time being. You will feel like a million dollars after you exercise and say to the external pressure: "Bring it on!!!".

We will see later how to make this temporary stress-free state of mind last. You will learn how to let go of the built-up negative emotions that are really at the cause of your response to external pressure.

I had to mention these two topics of food and exercise. But these are not what this book is all about. If we know what kind of food to eat and how to exercise, why aren't we all thin and happy? Let's be honest; the truth is, we already know exactly what we are supposed to do—in fact, with all the practice we've had, we probably know more about diets than the experts do. The question is, if it really is as easy as **'*just doing it*'**, why are we still overweight?

Knowing and not doing, is like not knowing at all. More than just food and exercise, we need a third key element.

So you know that our society has a problem. And more likely, you also know what to do about it. There's no shortage of information, books, magazines, Internet, friends, TV, recipes etc. So why isn't it working? Everybody knows to eat healthy and exercise. Even if you hire the best trainer in the world or the best Nutritionist there is, the trainer will not do the exercise for you. You still have to show up and do the work. Your best investment is in your own brain. It starts with your own motivation in order for you to execute what your trainer and nutritionist tell you to do. I am a fitness professional myself. I do strongly believe in working with qualifies professionals. I work with trainers myself. I am not saying you should not have a personal trainer or someone to work your meal plan with. What I am stressing here is the fact that your mind set is the key.

It is like you have been sitting on the passenger's seat of a car all your life, and even if you have lots of experience being in the car, it doesn't mean that you know how to drive.

KEY CONCEPTS:

OVERWEIGHT PROBLEM IN CANADA

54% of Canadians are overweight. Losing weight is not only about self-image. It contributes to overall health. See this book as a way to get off your pills.

PLATEAU

We get discouraged when our exercise efforts are no longer giving us results. As we progress and reach milestones in our fitness level, we need to re-evaluate our exercise routine and program ourselves.

PRESSURE vs STRESS

Pressure represents the external reasons why we create stress inside our body. Exercise can release the stress temporarily.

SOMETHING IS MISSING

Food and exercise are not the only factors to consider in order to lose weight.

CHAPTER 7

THE D.N.A. SYSTEM

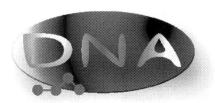

The structure of the system is quite simple. Pretend that you feel that you need to do some changes in your home. You are not quite happy with some of the rooms in your house. You have some company coming in a few months and you would like to do a few upgrades.

The first thing to do is to assess what you want to put your budget on first. What room will make the most impact and will give you the most satisfaction? That's the DESIRE part of the D.N.A. System: finding out what you want to work on and what is your vision of the new room.

Now let's say you have decided to make changes to your kitchen. Before installing the new cupboards, you first need to get rid of the existing ones. There is a demolition or a cleaning task to be done before putting the new cupboards in place. That is the NEW YOU part of the D.N.A. system. We clean up and get rid of old unwanted emotions, behaviours and beliefs and make room for what you want to implement in your life.

Once clear and empty, all you need is to fill up your kitchen with brand new cupboards and furniture, new paint, new floors, and whatever you have decided in your plan. The implementation of the desires to imprint them into your new you is the ACTUALIZE part of the D.N.A. system.

DISCIPLINE

I have prepared lots of opportunities for you to apply each concept as you go. The activities in this book are an adapted version of the processes that I use with my clients. As I am unable to be in the room with you, keep in mind that you may need to read an exercise a few times and master the steps before closing your eyes and fully immersing yourself in the exercise. I suggest that you read over all the questions in the exercise before starting, so that you know where you are going.

There will be different types of activities suggested. You will have your favorite ones. You may need to close your eyes and see what it looks like. You may choose to write. You may want to sit back and think about it. Just like with my clients, my auditory clients can be over the phone or Skype, and some clients want to physically be sitting in my office. I am lucky to be highly auditory so I can have a successful session with clients just over the phone without seeing them. (Depending on the processes that we are performing, of course, as some specific processes need me to see my clients' expressions.)

I recommend that you take these exercises seriously and take the time to do them with care. Do them when you are relaxed and have time to do them with purpose. First you will decide what you want your focus to be for the exercises, and what you want to work on. Be specific and focus on fixing one problem at a time.

KEY CONCEPTS:

D.N.A. SYSTEM

Desire. New You. Achieve.
Decide what you want. Make some room. Program the desires.

DISCIPLINE

Take the time to fully understand and perform the exercises that will be presented to you

CHAPTER 8

"D" FOR DESIRE

DESIRE VS WANT

Desire. When you ask people what they want or what they desire, most people respond with a negative affirmation telling what they don't want. They want to stop being fat. They want to stop feeling ashamed. They want to not feel tight in their clothes. Defining our desire is really important. It is like if you were to ask your interior designer who is helping you remodel your kitchen that you want them to paint the kitchen "not blue". Can you imagine the margin of error that is possible here? Even if you say that you would like the kitchen to be green. There are so many different types of green that it is necessary to be specific when it comes to what you want.

Now, what is the difference between what you want and what you desire? And why am I talking about desire? How much more effective are desires when it comes to setting up goals?

Let's pretend you hear a friend say: "I want to see that movie, it sounds good. I will see if I can get to it sometimes this week". Then another friend cuts the conversation and says: "Oh yes I heard about this movie, I absolutely have to see it, it sounds amazing! I have cleared my Tuesday night and I am going to the 6:50pm show". Which of the two friends do you think is more likely to see the movie? Which one seems to have the strongest desire to see it?

You want to make your *wanting to lose weight* into a compelling desire. Be on a mission to achieve your desire. When something is important to you, you make it happen. It is not like something on your to-do list. It is talking to you from the inside and you know you must do it. You are compelled and there is nothing that will get in your way. How amazing is that? Desires are happening at an unconscious level. Remember when we talked about your logical mind and your unconscious mind? You use your logical for your day-to-day and you tend to rely on it a lot. However, real change happens at an unconscious level. When your unconscious mind is set on something, it works in the background and executes the command. Can you imagine how great it will be when your wanting to lose weight becomes something so compelling that you naturally feel the need to fulfil it and will do everything that needs to be done? And this will happen at an unconscious level, behind the scenes. First, let's learn about your fascinating brain and its powerful complexity.

KEY CONCEPTS:

DESIRE VS. WANT

Desiring is more powerful than simply wanting. It is driven from the inside out, originating from the unconscious mind. Most people know what they don't want. A desire needs to be driven from the positive, from what they want.

CHAPTER 9

DEMAND

Demand. The first step is to know that you can actually demand your brain to accomplish your wishes. Whatever you tell your brain, it will happen. If you tell yourself you're fat, your brain will do that. It's like you're writing software for your brain. What are going to write on the software? How are you going to write down your own "you"? What are you going to be?

I often hear people say, "I wish I liked raw vegetables." Who told you that you don't like them? You did!! So you can tell your brain that you do like raw vegetables. You own your brain and you can write fresh software for your brain. Have you heard people say: "I am very bad with names. I wish I was good with names." My answer is always the same: Why aren't you? Who decided that you were bad with names? Who made the call?

Some people say: "I am a morning person" or "I am a night owl." They conditioned themselves to be that way and they believe it. If I need to stay up late, then I am an evening person and if I need to get up early, then I tell myself that I am a morning person. I can be both. Whatever is serving me. So if a thought is not serving you, change it! Just start believing you are good at remembering names, trust me, there is so much room in your brain, you remember a lot of things that you don't need, so why wouldn't there be room for a few extra names in there?

You probably all know a girl who can eat anything and she still stays thin. Do you know why? Because she thinks she can. Moreover, everyone is telling her: "You eat whatever you want and you still stay thin". She even gets the exterior reinforcement from friends on the outside world; her brain is listening to this. Every time she enters a building, her brain makes her go to the stairs because it wants to make her right about being thin, she probably never sees the close parking spot and always ends up parking at the end of the lot because her brain wants to make her right and walk more to stay thin, she probably pushes her plate away halfway through the meal, genuinely feeling full, easily, because her brain is telling her to do so.

The brain is very powerful. If you think that you can, you can. We all grew up with different patterns and we've been told these patterns for 20, 40 years. The good news is that we can rewrite these patterns. If you tell your brain you are skinny, it will make you stop eating earlier, it will make you avoid your 2nd serving and all the unwanted food. It will make you crave veggies and healthy stuff. You have to be careful how you talk to your brain. All you have to do is to demand. Do so and you will receive.

KEY CONCEPTS:

DEMAND

Your brain executes whatever you input in your *software*.

CHAPTER 10

DO NOT...

D o not... The words you use to make your demands to your brain matter. Whatever you focus on, you will get. What shows up in your mind if I tell you: "Do not make a mental picture in your head of Mickey Mouse dancing in a yellow Tuxedo." Did you see it? Of course you did. Even if I said: Do NOT visualize it. You get what you concentrate on. The reason why you saw it is because you had to process the information and then process the *do not* visualize it.

We asked the question: "Why do we sabotage ourselves?" Why is our brain doing this to us? If your body is a robot executing what the computer has been programmed for, there might be a software-programming problem in our brain. Who did the programming? You did! Every time you repeated to yourself that you were overweight.

Our brain is making us right. If somewhere in your mind you have a belief that you're fat and you have big thighs and you have a big belly, and if you have that belief and your brain hears it over and over, then your brain will make you right. If for the past 15 years we have been looking at ourselves in the mirror every day telling ourselves: "I have a big gut" or "I am fat" or "I have big thighs", you know all these discriminating thoughts we say and tell ourselves? Well the brain hears it loud and clear, and it does everything it can to make you right!!! We focus on not being fat or losing weight, so our brain hears *fat* and *extra weight*.

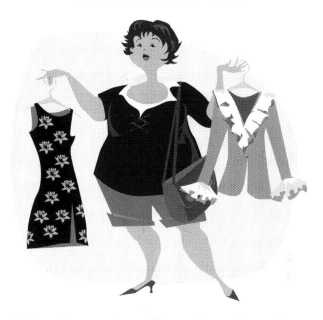

First of all, with a mind set of being fat, and your brain wanting to make you right, it will never really ask you to go for a workout or to reach for an apple or for raw veggies; it is doing everything it can to make you right and keep you fat, because that is what you are conditioned to be. You are thinking about yourself as a person with a big butt or a big belly or you think you are a size 12 or 14, or that you are 190lbs and that is the way it is.

Let's say that you kick butt for a while and you actually go for a workout and you start eating well and that you are actually starting to lose weight. Then your brain is panicking because it is saying: "oh no!... What is going on?... She is losing weight and she is supposed to be fat. What can I do...to make her right about being fat? Oh... here is a chocolate bar, I'm gonna make her eat that..." So we feel like we are sabotaging ourselves but the truth is that we are only making ourselves right about our thoughts.

You'll walk into the grocery store and your brain will see a bag of chips and make you right by making you buy it because you've said over and over that you are fat. Your brain will always make you right. 90% of our brain isn't used. It's very powerful and we don't want to underestimate its strength. We have to be really careful with the thoughts and words we put into our brain. We have to be careful what we want to be right about. Because no matter what, your brain will execute the thoughts you are putting in.

Here is an example. Three friends go to a movie together. They all came out of the movie and really enjoyed it. When they respectively got home, they told the story of the movie to their husbands. The first woman told her husband how this overweight lady performed a great life lesson in this movie where being unattractive and overweight didn't keep her from succeeding in life.

The second lady tells her husband how this movie was about a very funny lady, that appeared to not be really serious about work, got herself into the corporate world with a good paying position even though she wasn't working 24/7 and still had time for her children.

The third lady told her husband that the story was about a woman that defied the male-dominated corporate world and got to the top of her firm, ahead of the men that were applying for the promotions.

If I tell you that one of the friends is overweight, one of them is a family-oriented woman and the other one is a women's right advocate, do you know which one is which? Do you see how you get what you focus on? They all saw the same movie and somehow drew three different conclusions.

Another great example has probably already happened to you millions of times. You see a glass at the edge of the counter. You tell yourself that more likely it will fall on the floor and splash all over the whole kitchen. A moment later, you turn around and hit the glass "by accident". Or you see a report that you need to take to the office with you and you tell yourself: "I can't forget that tomorrow, if I do, I will be in big trouble at the office." The day after, you show up at the office and you forgot the report that you actually "programmed yourself to forget".

Have you ever opened the fridge, looking for the water jug, and not seen it at first glance? Then you said out loud: "I can 't find it" and you kept repeating it in your brain: "I can't see it, it is probably empty and in the sink or in the dishwasher. I can't find it". Then your spouse comes behind you and takes it right in front of your eyes. It was on the shelf, rye-level right in front of you but you had stopped your brain from seeing it. When you starting saying "I can't see it" You were making yourself right by not seeing it.

> *Whether you think you can or you can't, you're right either way.*
>
> *Henry Ford*

Be careful when you think. We tend to use the "do-not" way too often. We try to stay away from what we don't want instead of thinking with positive words. Focus on the right things and with the proper mind set and your brain will make it as easy as not shaving your face. What if you wanted to eat healthy things? What if you really wanted that? Can we fake it until we make it? In her study about physiological behaviour and psychological responses, social psychologist Amy Cuddy, social psychologist, comes to the conclusion that in fact, we can not only fake it until we make it, but we can fake it until we become it.

KEY CONCEPTS:

DO-NOT

Our mind has been conditioned for years to hate exercising and healthy food as we focus on the negative. Using do-not in our language is not serving our cause as much as we would like.

CHAPTER 11

DO IT WITH YOUR BODY AND THE MIND WILL FOLLOW

D o it. The mind and the body are connected. Each affects the other. Let's say for example, when you are tired, you curl up in a chair. Your brain associates the state of mind with the physical behaviour and then reverses the two: slumping in your chair can make you feel tired. The cause is now the effect and the effect is now the cause. Wouldn't it be great if we could just think about a state of mind that we want to feel and consciously enter it?

What if I tell you that I believe it is possible and that you all, at one point of your life did that? You know when you are having a bad day but it happens to be your 3 years old daughter's birthday? Then you immediately "force" yourself to enter a happy mood in order to avoid any suspicion from your kids? So that they don't realize that you are not feeling so well? Or when you feel down and you have to meet with your bosses' boss? You fake it and then before you know it, you are entering a different mood.

Amy Cuddy, social psychologist, demonstrated how our body language shapes who we are.

Body language is communication and interaction. It decides whom we ask out on a date, whom we choose to hire or promote. We are influenced by non-verbal communication, i.e. our feelings, our thoughts, our physiology, our non-verbal expressions of power and dominance. For example in the animal kingdom, we have all seen pictures of how animals expand, stretch themselves out and open up to show pride and power. The reverse is also true. When powerless, we make ourselves small.

In life, when interacting with others, we complement the other person's behaviour. If they are making themselves powerful, we tend to do the opposite.

Amy Cuddy responded to the question: "Can you fake it till you make it?" Can we choose to experience a behavioural outcome that makes us feel more powerful? We know that our non-verbal behaviours govern how other people think and feel about us. But the real question, in her research was: "Do our non-verbal actions govern how we think and feel about ourselves?"

Our mind changes our bodies and our bodies change our mind. In Cuddy's study, where the subjects needed to take a high power pose (standing with their chest up) or low power pose (sitting and curled up), their levels of cortisol (stress hormone) and testosterone (dominant hormone) changed significantly. The subjects in high power poses became more assertive, confident and comfortable. The subjects in the low power poses became really stress reactive and feeling kind of shut down.

Our nonverbal body language governs how we think and feel about ourselves. So yes, our bodies change our minds. Can power posing for a few minutes really change your life in meaningful ways? In Cuddy's study, high power posers had more presence. They were more passionate, enthusiastic, confident, captivating, comfortable and authentic. So our bodies change our minds, our minds change our behaviour and our behaviour changes our outcomes. Even when we say fake it till you make it, we don't really want to get the result and feel like a fraud or an imposter. So we don't only fake it till we make it but fake it 'til we become it! Tiny tweaks can lead to big changes.

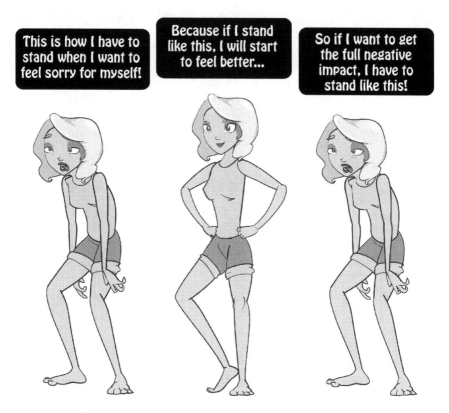

Knowing that your physiology is really impacting who you are, use this knowledge to your advantage. Just ask yourself at any given time: "How would I like to feel right now, what mood would I like to be in?" And proceed to enter the mood you want. Next time you are sitting on the couch, don't curl up, bring your hands behind your head, spread out, and be in a powerful pose so you will more likely be able to avoid the evening snacks.

When you do your grocery shopping, walk tall, shoulders back, no rounding your chest in with your shopping cart and your food choices will be better. Look confident. Put your body in a confident position. Give yourself this opportunity. Give yourself 5 seconds. Have you already made changes in the way you were standing or sitting as you are reading these words? Curling up might feel comfortable but if you are ready and know what you want, start looking like it. Change your position and look confident. Head up, chest lifted. You will get better results. You are in the process of gaining control over your body.

One of my favourite applications of this is the way I dress when I go grocery shopping. There are so many unhealthy choices jumping at me when I go to the store. Even at my favourite health food store, there are lots of "pretend-health-foods" that would like to put in my buggy. I dress myself in my best attire. I always make a point to dress up a bit for my trip to the grocery store. Funny right? But what do you think I will put in my cart when I am wearing nice clothes, heels on and feeling super self-confident? (Have you ever tried to walk in heels in a curled up position?). I tend to buy more unhealthy snacks when I am wearing a hoody and an old pair of jeans. Besides, I work from home and don't get much opportunity to wear my nice shoes so they are very happy to come out when we go grocery shopping. Walking in front of the baking department, I make a point to roll my shoulders back and lift my chin up and keep repeating to myself that I am fit and healthy and I will walk right past this section easily and with a big smile.

We will see other techniques later on how to get into a powerful mood when we get to the ACTUALIZE section of the D.N.A. system and introduce the techniques of anchoring and amplifying positive feelings.

KEY CONCEPTS:

DO IT WITH YOUR BODY AND THE MIND WILL FOLLOW

Mind and body are connected. You can use your physiology in order "trick" your mind into another state.

CHAPTER 12

DEDICATE

Dedicate. Imagine a professional tennis game where you could change a few variables: first, the number of balls used in the game and secondly, the number of opponents one should face at the same time. Pretend for a second that you are watching this tennis game where one of the best players in the world is playing against 10 other players that are firing at him 2 or 3 balls each. Can you see the chaos?

If people have too many balls in the air at once, they drop them. People who start new nutrition and exercise programs start off highly motivated and they have too many goals at once - cut the carbs, drink more water, go for a run, go to the gym, get divorced, quit smoking, etc. If you try to address everything at once, it doesn't work. You get overwhelmed, which leads to depression and feeling bad. Your brain reminds you of the negative feelings when it hears the words diet, nutrition, or exercise.

The following exercise will help you with dedicating your energy to one goal. Just like our previous example of choosing which room you will renovate in your house. By doing one thing at a time, you will have a much greater chance of getting positive results than if you try and change everything at once.

If you prefer to write your answers separately, remember that you can download my free Think Yourself Thin workbook at www. dnalifecoaching.com

DIVIDE

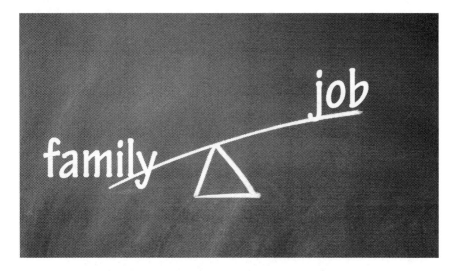

You are now invited to divide your life into eight segments. While you may think that your life is separated into two - work and family - there are lots of other areas that influence your life. There seems to be a misconception of the word BALANCE. Most people think that there are two components of a life: Family and Job. Isn't it true that everybody talks about finding balance between these two things?

Think of your life as a pie chart with many slices such as career, love life, family, health, etc. It might be that one area of your life (one slice) doesn't make you happy and this will interfere with your weight loss plan. Rate each area of your life out of 10 as to whether or not you are happy in these areas. If you see an area that's only 3 or 4 out of 10, you might chose to fix this area before you start your weight loss and nutrition plan. Work on one area at a time. If a wheel isn't balanced, the ride will be bumpy. Remember to write the numbers that you feel are the best representation for yourself. Avoid thinking about what others would think of what your number should be.

For instance, I had a client once who did not have a significant other. For the part of the wheel *Love and Romance*, she gave herself a 10. She was absolutely fine with being by herself. That is what was okay for her, in her representational system. If I had asked her mother, the mother would have probably given her a 1 out of 10 for *Love and Romance*. It is not about how other people feel about each segment. It is about you. Same thing with a client who was making $25,000 per year giving herself 8 out of 10 for *Money*. That was all she needed in her own model of reality.

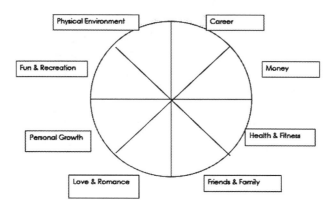

Feel free to rename the segments if the label doesn't fit in your life and you would rather see something else there. Once you have given a number to each segment, make a line representing the number and colour the area from the centre of the wheel up to the line. That will look like this:

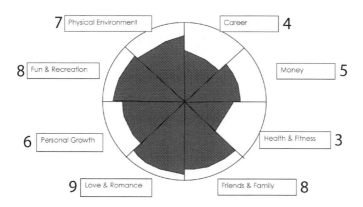

Pretend that you are a truck and that you roll on these wheels. Do you think that the road might be a little bumpy? The bumps in our journey are caused by unbalances in the different areas of our life. It is because of these differences that deceptions and dissatisfaction are troubling us.

I once had a client that filled out the wheel and gave herself a three in all the segments but one where she had a 7. This was a recent 7. A few months back, she would have given herself a three in all the segments. She told me that she had been in a rut for years. Her ride was smooth though. She had a constant three. That made the wheel quite small and she was not going very fast but she was not even noticing that all the areas of her life were not satisfying because there was no bump in the road to make her realize the differences. When she suddenly improved one part of her life and got a seven, she realized she had been missing out on everything else and it gave her the trigger she needed and that is when she found my website. We worked on each segment one at a time and after addressing only 3 segments, somehow, all segments had improved. They are all inter-connected.

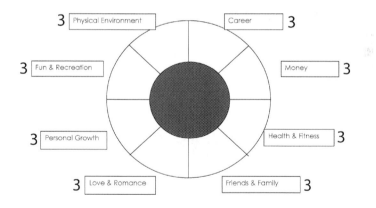

Now think about your results and have a closer look at each segment. Try to identify the connections between each and every one of them. Because this book is about weight loss, let's focus on the Health and Fitness segment of the wheel. What other segment is connected to it? Let's say that if you work on your job, you will be able to free up some time to go to the gym. Or if you get out of an abusive relationship, you might find the self-confidence you need to make better food choices. Or if you take more time for friends or personal growth, you will reduce stress, which makes you overeat. You may have a much more pressing matter to address before being able to focus on your weight-loss.

- Some areas influence others. Which area(s) of your wheel influence(s) your weight loss?
    - ○ _____
    - ○ _____
    - ○ _____
- Which one do you want to address first?
    - ○ _____

Now that you have identified which area of the balance wheel you want to work on, you are now ready to determine what you want and what is your desired outcome regarding this area of your life.

Once you go through the D.N.A. system with that area of your life, you can start over and chose another area. You can also choose to re-define and create a more focused wheel that addresses all areas of weight-loss. For example, you could have the following segments and work on one of them at a time: Activity level, Eating Out, Snacking, Grocery Shopping, Meal Planning, Cardio-vascular training, Strength training, beverages & water intake.

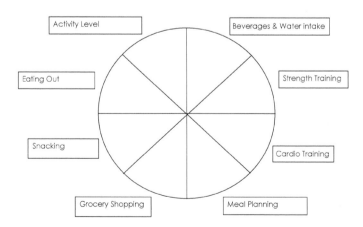

KEY CONCEPTS:

DEDICATE

Focus on one thing at a time

DIVIDE

Use the exercise to chunk down the pieces and focus on one problem at a time. Observe how all areas of your life are connected and which one have an effect on weight-loss.

CHAPTER 13

DETERMINE

D etermine. Now, it is time to determine what you want. I know you have more likely done this millions of times. You may even be tired of promising yourself, once again, that this will be the year that you finally lose the weight. How many times have you been on a diet, given up, tried again, and lost the weight, only to put it all back on again? Would you feel better and happier about yourself if you lost maybe 10 lbs, maybe 30 lbs, maybe even more? Here we go again! Have you ever lost weight and gained it back? Yes, that happens right? And the question that I want you to ask yourself right now is: Is it necessary for you to lose weight? Did your doctor tell you that you need to lose weight? What is it going to do for you if you lose weight? It's really important that you know that. This book will teach you how to lose the weight and how to keep it off and how to love yourself and love what you see in the mirror. That's the most important thing. It is about feeling great about yourself and not about what others could think or want you to do. It is about YOU first.

DETERMINE THE INTENTION BEHIND THE DESIRE OF LOSING WEIGHT

Most behaviours start with good intentions. Even the teenager who takes on smoking to belong and feel the part, even criminals usually start out with good intentions and then go downhill from there. Behaviour is always valuable somewhere at some time. Anger is useful when someone is under attack. Anger out of context may be an attempt to get people to understand. It may not however be useful or gain the desired result.

When you eat a burger that you shouldn't have, and you didn't really want to eat it, there was a positive intention behind your behaviour. Perhaps you wanted to recreate the memories that you had on that fun summer weekend when you went away with your friends and enjoyed many BBQ's. If you had thought about the intention behind the behaviour, maybe you would have realized that all you wanted was to remember that fun summer. If you had, you could have found another way to fulfil that intention - a way that doesn't involve calories. You could have picked up the phone and called one of the friends that were there with you. You could have sent out an invitation to organize another trip with your friends. You could have looked at pictures of the party. Instead, you ate a burger and soon enough, your brain associated that act with emotions of fun with your friends. The next thing you know it becomes a habit and burgers are a huge part of your life. But really, only your friends are that important, not the burgers themselves.

Finding the intention behind the behaviour becomes very relevant when it comes to getting rid of a bad habit. One of my clients wanted to quit smoking, and all on his own he decreased to one cigarette per day but was unable to completely quit. It turned out, after asking the right questions during coaching sessions, that he had not yet accepted the fact that his father had passed away. His father was a smoker so the cigarette was connecting him to his memories with his father. He did not want to let him go. Finding the intention behind the unwanted behaviour helps to find other ways to fulfil that positive intention. Now instead of having his one cigarette at night (the unwanted behaviour) he takes out the photo album and looks at photos of his father so that he can connect and honour his memory. He has been smoke free for almost 8 years and is now running half-marathons.

Our cravings are often connected to deeper memories and triggered by our senses. We all know that certain smells remind of us of certain things. Mom's cooking always made us feel good. Have you ever walked into a movie theatre or a bakery? You can smell the popcorn or the fresh baked goods and immediately, the cravings start. Find the reason behind the craving and then find a different way to fulfil that craving. If you miss your mom, call her or look at some pictures. You don't need to eat a whole chocolate cake because it makes you think about her. You still can think about her and love her without having to sabotage your health over it!

Here is another great example that shows how finding the intention behind the behaviour can help modify the behaviour. I had a client once who moved to a new city. All of a sudden she kept buying a certain type of chocolate bar and eating it and she couldn't understand why. Every day she needed her chocolate bar. She never used to like chocolate and it was never a problem before even when she actually used to work for the manufacturer of that particular chocolate bar. (Which was quite ironic, a chocolate sales rep that doesn't like chocolate.) So why was she all of a sudden eating chocolate? What had changed? She called me and said: "Nathalie, you have to help me, I am eating chocolate every day and I am going out of my mind! I never used to like chocolate! What is going on?" After a few sessions, we realized that she missed the life she had when she was working for the chocolate company. She had moved and was now alone in her new city. Eating chocolate was her way of coping with feeling lonely and missing her friends. She didn't really want the chocolate bar; she wanted to be with her old friends. Now, instead of eating chocolate bars, she phones or connects with her friends on email or Facebook, which is a much healthier way to fulfil the intention behind the behaviour. She has gotten back to her healthy eating habits and is now in Australia and still keeps in touch with her friends on the web.

In the activities below, I will ask lots of questions about your intentions. You now know the reason why going deeper than the simple: "I want to lose weight because I want to be slim" will increase your success rate.

DETERMINE YOUR EXPECTATION WITH THIS BOOK

As you just read, the intention behind the behaviour is connected with the solution to fixing our problem. Therefore, it is always good to understand what we want and what is our objective when we do something.

The first exercise is to write down what you want from this book. You have identified the area that you want to work on. I am using examples related to weight-loss in the below exercise. You may want to apply them to another area if, for example, you have decided to work on your career first.

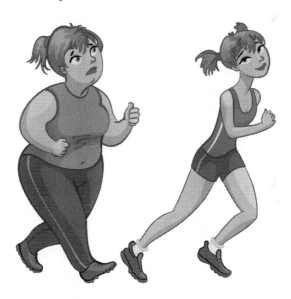

Now, pretend you are on the phone with me and this is just like your intake interview. You are describing your problem to me and telling why you feel that you need help. What do you want with this book? Allow the first thing that pops in your head to be the answer. What do you want from this book? This can be done very quickly. It could be "I want to lose weight" or "I want to eat vegetables and love them", "I hate running and I want to start loving it", "I am intrigued by this Thinking Yourself Thin idea and I want to know what this is all about", or "I am a wellness professional and I am always interested in reading new things that I could bring to my own clients".

When you know why, it's easier to lose weight. It's important to know why you want to lose weight. What is the first thing that comes to your mind? Do you want to have fun exercising, fit into your jeans, or bend over easily to tie your shoes, stand on one foot to shave your legs in the shower, feel great on a first date, look fabulous in your wedding dress, live a longer and stress-free life? What is your outcome? What do you expect?

An example of a participant in one of my seminars:

> "I want to stop yo-yo-ing. I have a 40 year pattern of gaining weight over the winter and then having to lose it before the summer. It's a huge struggle."

This person has developed a pattern that she has learned and she became really good at that pattern until it became her regular routine. She has a habit of gaining and losing weight. In order to break that habit, there are some specific processes that you will learn soon to easily replace the old habit by a new better one. We will see these techniques later. For now, let's rephrase that positive outcome into something more positive: *"I want to keep the weight off once I have come to my healthy weight* (instead of stop yo-yo-ing). *I used to struggle with the winter and now I have new techniques and tools that are making me stay thin over the winter and feel great all year long. I have developed a new habit of being healthy and I am becoming unconsciously competent at it."*

I am actively reading this book in order to:

_____

_____

_____

_____

How do you know you need to lose weight?

"I know I want to lose weight because nothing fits me anymore and I keep going up a size every year".

_____

_____

How long have you wanted to lose weight?

"It started after the birth of my second child."
"It has always been on my mind for as long as I can remember"

_____

_____

What happened the first time you went on a diet?

"I lost 15 pounds in no time and gained it all back a few months later"

_____

_____

What else has happened since then? What changed in your life? Did you move? Did you get a new job? Did you meet someone? Did you have kids? Did someone close to you pass? Is everything the same? Is there anything worth mentioning that could be linked to your weight-loss unfortunate results?

_____

_____

What is the relationship between these events and your current situation?

"After I had my kids, I changed my priorities to serve the needs of my children and stopped exercising"

_____

_____

Think about your parents, siblings, friends and partner. What is the relation between this person (mother, father, brother, friend, etc.) and your current weight situation?

"My mother used to bake for us when we were sad or upset. Somehow, I now have the reflex to revert to baking goods as a pick-me-up solution."

_____

_____

Is there anything relevant about your childhood in relation to your weight?

"I have many siblings and we had to eat fast in order to make sure there would still be enough food left if we wanted seconds."

_____

_____

What is there to lose?

Once you have reached your weight-loss goal, what will be missing that is currently present? What is in your life now that will not be there anymore once you've lost the weight?

For example:

"I won't feel self loathing anymore"
"I won't be exhausted all the time"
"The comments from people who are telling me I am fat will be gone"
"The shame will be gone"
"The camouflage clothing will go"
"I will lose the habit of fixing up my shirt to avoid showing the fat rolls every time I sit down"

_____

_____

_____

What is there to gain?

Did you notice how easy it is to say what we don't want? Now, instead, what do you want? A lot of people say: "I don't want to be fat". Can you turn this from a negative to a positive? What would you like instead? Answer what you want, not what you don't want.

What do you want to change about your weight? Be specific.

"I want to go back to a realistic size 8 as I used to be that size in my adult life." *"I specially want the extra weight around my weight to be gone as this is where my organs are being squished the most by the extra fat and losing weight will make all the systems in my body work better. My digestion will be improved as well as my cardio-vascular ability, my skin will glow and my flexibility improved. I will be able to bend over easily."*

_____

_____

_____

More precision please

Now we can expand the intention a bit more. Use the next exercise to give more substance to your goal. Which colour is the bikini you will buy? Where are you going to go shopping for it? Which beach are you going to? What feelings exactly are you going to feel? What will people tell you? What will you tell yourself when you look at the mirror?

There's probably a reason for you to want to lose weight. Maybe there is more than one reason. And whatever those reasons are, imagine you have finally lost the weight. What will be present in your life that is currently missing? Beyond the appearance, what else is there to gain with your weight loss? What is the intention behind the behaviour?

Visualize yourself being thin. What does that do for you? Does it empower you, does it give you self-confidence, and does it give you energy? What does it do?

Example of one of my clients: *I want to lose weight and feel healthy and beautiful.*

The portion *'feeling healthy and beautiful'* is perfect in this sentence. The words *'lose weight'* are not really an end result. It is an action that will lead to feeling healthy and beautiful. But losing weight in itself is not that precise and does not generate feelings. So when you elicit your positive outcome, it is necessary to ask yourself what you really want beyond the behaviour and go further into the beliefs and the values. We will see the differences between behaviour and values and beliefs later on in this book. This sentence should be instead: *I want to feel healthy and beautiful.*

What will come into your life that's currently missing?

For example:

"I will have more self-confidence"
"I will meet a boyfriend when I lose weight"
"I will go skating with my son"
"I will run with my dog"
"I will shop for new clothes confidently "

_____

_____

_____

How will you know you have achieved your outcome in reading this book? What needs to happen when you finish reading that will prove that you have achieved your outcome? For example, let's pretend your outcome was to wear a bikini on the beach this summer. For some people, the moment that they are in the change room at the store buying the bikini, liking the reflection in the mirror, would be the moment that they know they have achieved their goal. For some others, the moment they lay on a lounge chair at the beach in their bikini would be the decisive moment. For some others, the moment they go for a walk on the beach and feel great about it would be it. So in your case, what is the moment that you will know that you have achieved your goal in reading the book?

_____

_____

KEY CONCEPTS:

DETERMINE

Every behaviour has a positive intention in some context. Knowing this intention helps you understand the unconscious reasons for you to want something in particular.

Knowing what you want and writing your expectations & desires will set the tone for the unconscious mind to open the gate to new possibilities.

Asking yourself what you want, what you don't want and making your goal precise and compelling will start making it real in your head.

Going over the elements and people in your life that have affected your present situation is helpful to understand what led you to where you are now.

CHAPTER 14

DARE

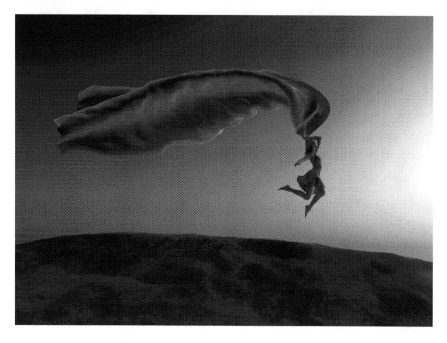

D are. The first exercise has opened your mind to finding out what you want. Now it is time to create a compelling image of yourself achieving your goal. When you do the exercise, remember to be daring and asking for the best possible outcome.

Remember I mentioned the client I coached who wanted to find a boyfriend? She had pictured a perfect outcome and actually met a man that had everything on her list. All she had imagined was there. Only one problem: once she got it, she thought about something else she would have liked to be on the list. She called me asking what to do. First of all, as mentioned, there is no failure, only feedback. This was great news. It meant that it had worked. She had been able to find what she wanted. I told her to do the process again and add on to her outcome the things that she had left out. Her first reaction was: "Well, I feel bad, this guy is quite nice, maybe he will do for a while, I don't know if I want to meet someone else right now... what will happen if I make a new list and then meet the guy that has everything? Then, I will have to drop my present boyfriend and I would feel really bad." Isn't that funny how she was now in full awareness of her power and was afraid to dare and to want more for her life because she was in a satisfying situation?

I also mentioned earlier in this book that everything and everybody are stepping stones towards something else. We grow, we evolve and we change. The first boyfriend she found was great. He served a great role in her life. He gave her the self-confidence to realize she could have more. She deserved more. Without him, she may not have found out. He was a stepping-stone towards what was coming next for her. She would not be serving him by staying with him because she, also, was more likely a stepping stone in his life. They stayed together for a while and she decided to make another list to see what could happen. She found another guy and they are now travelling the world together. As it turned out, she dared and it happened.

Remember to include as much as you want on your wish list. Although I made the analogy of the kitchen renovations, this is quite different in the way that for your dreams, you have an open budget. No restrictions. Give yourself lots of choices. You always want to aim to increase choice in your life.

If you can dream it, you can do it.

Walt Disney

Create more choices and more opportunities for yourself. As people get better strategies, they will use them. If you get a tool, you will use it.

In any field, the top people in that field are those who have the most variety in their behaviour. They have choices of behaviour that their colleagues don't.

Any time you limit your behavioural choices you give others the competitive edge. If you are able to respond to any situation in a variety of ways, you are more likely to get your outcome.

When you write your positive outcome, make sure you include lots of choices. Make sure you plan to be flexible and adaptive and that you program your brain to like many different types of exercise and a variety of food. Aim for the least restrictions as possible.

For example, I try to stay away from labels like 'vegetarian' or 'vegan' or 'dairy free' or 'gluten free.' Of course I chose to eat healthy. I don't eat meat, nor dairy, nor gluten. I only eat steal cut oats and quinoa as far as grains and starch are concerned and most of my meals are plant based and raw. But I would never consider myself a vegan or a raw food person because I think it only restricts me. What if I go to a friend's house and they are serving meat or chicken? I will politely have a small bite and most likely I won't die from it. Do I choose that on a regular basis? No. But what if I am on the go and forgot to carry my shake with me or my nuts or my veggie sticks? Or I run out because I have been gone longer than planned? I need to be able to get something on the go and if it is a veggie pita (even though I don't eat bread) then I will eat it with great pleasure and not sweat about it.

I think diets are restrictions and I prefer to adopt a lifestyle rather than a diet. Having choice is better than no choice and this applies to nutrition as well. It can also be quite loudly applicable if you recently had a visit with your doctor and he told you that you are suffering from high cholesterol or need to cut your sugar or salt intake. Again, then, you don't have choice and you are making changes for the wrong reasons.

Eliciting a well-formed outcome on paper is a great way to start the programming process. I'm sure you have heard of SMART (specific, measurable, achievable, realistic, timely) Goals. This method is similar in some ways.

You have probably also heard of "the list" that we do when we want something or "vision boards". These are great when they are correctly elicited and followed by the next steps necessary to bring them to life. Let's remember that these vision boards and smart goals are only ONE section of the D.N.A. system. In this section, we are figuring out what we want. We still have to do the clean-up with the NEW YOU section and then apply the concepts after in the ACTUALIZE section.

You have already defined what you wanted in the previous exercise. Here are some questions to guide you into making this into a well-formed outcome. As a reminder, your unconscious mind loves repetition. If you are faced to a question and you feel you have already responded, take a deep breath and ask your unconscious mind to give you the answer. The repetition is voluntary. Even if your logical mind thinks that you have already responded to this, keep going and go through all the questions.

What is your current situation? Where are you at now regarding your goal?

Are you starting your weight loss journey? Have you lost weight before?

What do you want? You can use a recap of everything you discovered in the previous exercise to write down the perfect success in the context you are considering. State what you want in positive terms, i.e. what do you want, and what do you want it to do? Where do you want it? When do you want it? Example: 'I want to be, do or have X'. If the answer forms as 'I do not want...' then ask, 'What do I want instead of...' For example, you would write: I am feeling great in my clothes. It is my wedding day and I am in the best shape of my life. I weight 135 lbs and I feel fabulous!

_____

_____

_____

Use your senses and add details. What will you see, hear and feel when you have it?

In this section, you will make a mental image of your outcome. Add on all the details you need to make it more compelling. Remember that your brain can process information so much faster that you can write or express it on paper. This question will be done in your head. See your outcome happening. See it as if it is happening now. Add on more details based on your senses. What else do you see? What do you hear? What are you saying in your head? How do you feel? Place that image on a giant screen and turn the dial up. Add on everything you need to make it nicer, brighter, more compelling, dare to dream everything you want to be part of this picture. See yourself as a third person looking at you in the picture. Once you have seen everything you needed to see, heard everything you needed to hear and felt everything you needed to feel, take the picture and insert it in your timeline in your future. It is like placing the picture as a to-do list for your unconscious mind. You are telling your unconscious mind that this is what will happen in your future. Your unconscious mind will keep working on achieving the result as it was just told that this was going to happen. Your brain doesn't know the difference between reality and fiction. It just executes what you tell it that is going to happen.

What will you accept as evidence that you have achieved your outcome? What evidence will you accept that lets you know when you have the outcome? Ensure that your evidence criteria are described in sensory based terms i.e.: That which you can see, hear and/or touch that proves to you and/or third parties that you have done what you set out to do. You will see on the scale the number you have looking for? You will buy a pair of pants in size 6? You will start craving apples and love your coffee without sugar?

What will that do for you?

Remember the secondary benefits? The intention behind the behaviour? What will achieving your outcome do for you? What else will that bring you?

Are you the one initiating this and do you have control over what you are asking?

Let's take for example the list that one of my clients made of her special desired soul mate. She had made the list of how she wanted him to be. How she wanted him to look, what she wanted him to do and how she wanted him to dress. The problem here is that the list can never be about what you want. It has to be about YOU. So instead of writing: "I want him to be tall, brown hair and have a great job, she re-wrote her list in using herself instead of him. She wrote instead: "I find him very attractive, I am happy with him, he makes me feel secure as he has a great job, he tells me that he loves me, etc." We can program our own brain to how we want to feel, what we want to see and hear, but we cannot program somebody else's brain.

Is it under your control, i.e. can you, personally do, authorize or arrange it? Anything outside your control is not 'well formed'. Registering for a fitness class is within your control. So is hiring a personal trainer. Asking your employer for time off is not. The time off will only become well formed if it is granted. For example, it is hard to predict that your family will also be losing weight with you. It would be a mistake to state that on paper. Just like it would be a mistake to predict the weather. Your well-formed outcome is about you and you have to be able to control it.

Is it achievable? Is it possible for a human being to achieve the outcome? If someone has done it, then in theory you can do it, too. If you are the first, find out if it is possible. I do believe in the power of the brain and I believe that anything is possible, however, if your goal is to jump off a cliff and take off flying, you might want to re-write your goal. If your goal is to lose 200 lbs in a month, you might want to reconsider putting something reasonably achievable in there. It must be something that is humanly possible, and then you could potentially do it. Your outcome has to be within the realm of human capability. If it is doable, then your brain can make you dream it and can make you right.

Are the costs and consequences of obtaining this outcome acceptable? Ensure that the outcome is worth the time, outlay and effort involved in achieving it, and that impact on third parties or the environment is accounted for. Your dream has always been to open your own aesthetics school but if you did so, you would never see your children as you would be working every weekend. How about you plan for it and wait a few years once your kids are off to school before doing it? Would that be worth it then? What are your values telling you?

_____

_____

_____

Do you have all the resources you need to achieve your outcome? Do you have or can you obtain all the resources, both tangible and intangible that you need to achieve your outcome? Resources include knowledge, beliefs, objects, premises, people, money, and time. Do you need to read some books on nutrition? Do you need to subscribe to some podcasts or health website or blogs that will feed you with information during your weight loss journey? Do you need to hire a personal trainer that will create a specific program for you?

_____

_____

_____

The following questions are really important. I just want to remind you here that your unconscious loves repetition and that answering every single question is part of the process.

What will you gain if you have it? *I will gain self-confidence*

_____

_____

What will you lose if you have it? *I will lose the heavy feeling that I carry around*

_____

_____

What will happen if you get it? *I will be happy with myself*

What won't happen if you get it? *I won't be ashamed of myself anymore*

What will happen if you don't get it? *I will continue feeling depressed and unhappy*

What won't happen if you don't get it? *I won't be able to run with my kids if I don't get it*

If you could have it now, would you take it? Are all costs and consequences of achieving your outcome, including the time involved, acceptable to you and anyone else affected by it? This is known as ecology. Consider the costs, consequences, environmental and third party impact of having the outcome. Let's say you have wanted to separate from your spouse, as you believed your relationship was going down the drain. If you could be divorced right now, would you take it? Let's say the year of separation was over, the paperwork was done, the house was sold, you had moved into a new place and all was final. Would you be happy now? Would you take it if it were handed on a silver platter to you right now?

Does your outcome fit with you?

If you were to achieve your outcome, would that be in line with your personality, your family system and your overall values? Does that fit with who you are? Are you 5 foot tall wanting to become a professional basketball player? Or do you have the shape of a football player with strong athletic features and want to weigh less than a hundred pounds? If in order to get to your goal, for example, you had to leave town for 3 years and not see your children and family. Is that acceptable to you?. Respond honestly to the question. Everybody has different values. Make sure that your outcome fits with yourself and your values.

When and how do you want your outcome?

Decide on a realistic time frame to achieve your goal. What is your deadline, where was the image deposited on your timeline? How will this happen?

Nothing happens unless first a dream

Carl Sandburg

It is now time to write the software that will reprogram your brain. Write your full daring desire.

Start with your full name and then write yourself new software:

My name is .... and.....

For example, if it is your daughter's wedding in July, your positive outcome can be:

"I am looking great and feeling great in my mother of the bride's dress that I am wearing at my daughter's wedding in July. I am at peace as everything is ready and planned perfectly. We have time to enjoy ourselves and take full advantage of this perfect day where love is embracing everybody. People are telling me how fabulous I look. I feel proud and happy with my body and all the work I did to reach my weight-loss goals. I can see my daughter being at her best and tremendously happy. I can smell the scents of the flowers on this gorgeous July day and I have a wonderful feeling going through my body that will keep me happy for years to come."

Here are a few more examples:

"I can eat whatever I want. I want good healthy food for myself. I eat the right portions for myself and it's easy for me to stop eating when I've had enough. I exercise easily and I love it. I have made a habit of eating well and exercising and I am unconsciously competent at it. I can wear whatever I want and it gives me so much self-confidence to know that I can go out and buy new clothes and everything fits great. I hear people tell me how great I look and I feel amazing. I love what I see in the mirror now and I love myself."

"I love my new life. I have successfully changed my old behaviours into new habits that are serving me. Eating healthy food and exercising is natural and easy for me. I can breeze through life in a light way and I have the self-confidence to introduce myself to highly intelligent, attractive and motivated people like me. I am happy to be surrounded by positive influences that keep me on track with my new choices. I always find ways to stay motivated and inspired."

Once you have written your statement, place copies of your statement all over your house, in every room and in your car. Write everything as if it's happening in the present, as if it's happening right now.

My name is _____ and I _____

_____

_____

_____

_____

_____

_____

_____

_____

_____

_____

_____

You can add to your statement as time goes by. It is always good to keep it updated and make sure that your statement changes and evolves with yourself and your changing desires.

Read this statement several times a day and at least once out loud so that your brain hears it out loud. There is a popular belief that it takes 21 days to re-create new neuro-pathways through the brain, to create the new habit. This statement came from Doctor

Maxwell Maltz in the 1950s from a research with patients that were receiving plastic surgery. It would take them in average 21 days in order to get us to their new nose for example[4]. As you can realize now, this research, although quite popular is quite dated. I prefer to follow the results of Doctor Phillippa Lally which conducted a research in 2009 with volunteers who chose an eating, drinking or activity behaviour to carry out daily in the same context for 12 weeks. The study published in the European Journal of Social Psychology reported that the average time to reach automaticity for performing an initially new behaviour was 66 days.[5]

So read it for at least 2 months (66 days). If you catch yourself thinking negative thoughts, ask yourself why? Turn your negative thoughts into positive thoughts. It took years for you to get where you are now, it might take a few months to reset your brain and create new habits. I will teach you more about neuro pathways in the NEW YOU section of the D.N.A. System. We will anchor your positive outcome later in the ACHEIVE section. For now, the first step is to tell your brain what you DESIRE.

Once you are well wired and well programmed, your brain will always continue working on it, whether you are conscious about it or not. You know how sometimes you think about a song and you just cannot get the title of the song, you can't seem to remember it? Then you stop thinking about it and it comes back 2 hours later? Well, in fact, you think that you stopped thinking about it but your brain (the 90% of the brain that we don't use) kept working on it, it never stopped looking for the title as you had ordered it to do so when you said: "I will remember it later". So a brain that is well wired will always deliver.

I will give you a concrete example of a well-wired brain. Mine. I think that I am the luckiest person in the world and I always get what I want. A few years ago we were in Mexico with a group. Our

---

[4] http://jamesclear.com/new-habit
[5] https://www.ucl.ac.uk/news/news-articles/0908/09080401

friends were all going to a restaurant at night. They had reserved for the 10 of them and we wanted to join them so we tried to get the reservation changed to 12 and even though I used my Spanish to negotiate with the waiter, nothing worked! They said they simply could not accommodate 12 of us. So my husband and I had to go eat somewhere else that night. Let me tell you that I was ticked off... It was impossible. How could this be happening? I always get what I want! Well, the day after at the hotel, everybody was sick with food poisoning. I am programed to be lucky and healthy and my brain knew all this because I believe somewhere in there, a portion of it can tell the future, so there you have it! If you are well programmed, you don't need to think about it anymore. Your brain works for you and makes things happen for you.

Another funny example is that I believe that I have a parking fairy. I always get the best parking spot! Even after over 10 years with my husband he still gets ticked off about it and sometimes he says, "Well, where is your parking fairy now?" And I say, "Keep going, somebody will pull out," and sure enough, somebody backs up from their spot and I get the parking spot. I believe that our brain is THAT powerful! That somehow while I am on my way my brain sends a message to the lady in the store telling her it is time to go home because she needs to leave in order for me to get her spot.

Some people call it the Universe, some people call it God, everybody has a different name for when these things happen. I just like to think that it is just another example of how powerful is our brain.

KEY CONCEPTS:

DARE

Complete the questionnaire and elicit a positive outcome that will satisfy your desires. Once you have elicited your outcome, continue to read it and keep letting your brain know that this is what you want.

CHAPTER 15

"N" FOR NEW YOU

New You. The second step of the D.N.A. System is to make some room to implement what you just elicited. Your unconscious mind has already started to work on your desires. Your outcome has been planted and now we need to make sure that there is plenty of space for your outcome to grow. Just like in our original example, in order to get the new dream kitchen, you need to do some demolition and get rid of the out-dated cupboards.

Rest assured that all of the methods and processes that I use with my clients are light and effortless. When working with a new client, I sometime can sense their stress level rising when I mention this part. They think that I will psychoanalyse their past and they will have to re-live their negative experiences and dig through the dirt and cry and suffer until the demons have been exorcised. Please. Relax. You are not about to do any of this. This is the best part. The clearing section is empowering, insightful, cleansing and most of all, easy! Let me introduce you the main source of my techniques: Neuro-Linguistic Programing.

KEY CONCEPTS:

NEW YOU

You have elicited your desire and now is time to make some room in order for your outcome to have space to be implemented

CHAPTER 16

NEURO-LINGUISTIC PROGRAMMING

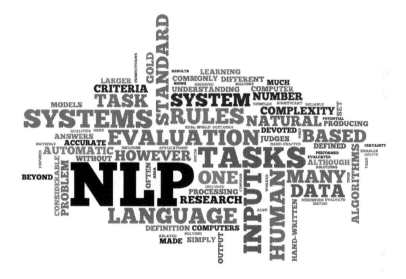

euro-Linguistic Programming (NLP) is an approach to communication, personal development, and psychotherapy created by Richard Bandler and John Grinder in California, USA in the 1970s. *Neuro* refers to the mind and how we organize our mental life. *Linguistic* is about language, how we use it and how it affects us. *Programming* is about our sequences of repetitive behaviour and how we act with purpose.[6] NLP is about the connection between our thoughts, speech and actions, which are what connects us to others, the world and to the spiritual dimension.

---

[6] *Way of NLP* - Joseph O'Connor & Ian McDermott

Bandler and Grinder claim that the skills of exceptional people can be "modelled" using NLP methodology, and then those skills can be acquired by anyone.[7]

Anthony Robbins, a very famous NLP Master Practitioner created this definition of NLP: The science to reprogram your own brain.

Lynn Robinson, my Master NLP Trainer from the Robinson Group, defines NLP as the model of excellence and the science of language.

I also like how Stepheni Smith and Peter Freeth defined NLP in their book NLP Practitioner Basics that you need to know to practice NLP: "NLP is a toolkit to reorganise our experience so that they can be useful in the future."

NLP bases its processes on different basic beliefs and assumptions that guide and have guided the development of NLP. They are not necessarily true, but produce useful results. Beliefs are usually self-fulfilling. If we believe someone doesn't like us, our defensive manner can make this a reality. If we believe we can master a skill, we persevere until we do. We call them presuppositions because you presuppose that they are true and act on them. If you act as if they were true, you will find yourself, your life and your interactions with others become more effective, interesting, satisfying and enriching.

KEY CONCEPTS:

NEURO-LINGUISTIC-PROGRAMMING

NLP is the science that teaches you how to reprogram your brain using linguistic.

---

[7] *The Ultimate Introduction to NLP* - Richard Bandler.

CHAPTER 17

NEED

N eed. You have already been introduced earlier to a few NLP presuppositions. "There is no failure, only feedback", "mind and body are connected" and "there is a positive intention behind all behaviours" were already explained to you. Here are a few more of my favourite presuppositions.

PEOPLE HAVE ALL THE RESOURCES THEY NEED TO SUCCEED.

This opens up possibilities. By resources, I mean the internal responses and external behaviours needed to get a desired response. Often people have resources that they haven't considered or are available in other contexts. Maybe you know someone who shows good leadership skills at work but can't manage his or her children. A lot of my clients are wondering why they can be so polite with strangers and yet, be so abrupt when it comes to talking to their spouse or partner. Why is that that we can have a skill - patience in this example - and not use it? If you have the skill you have it. It is like being pregnant. You cannot be pregnant just sometimes. You are or you aren't. When you have a skill, you have it. Period. So if you can be patient with strangers, you can be patient with your partner. It is just a matter of re-wiring our brains.

All the capability is within us and is waiting to be discovered. Let's stop limiting ourselves. We all have what we need. Everybody has the internal brainpower and the capability if they put their mind to it. You don't have to wait.... you don't have to say, "When I get this, then I will do that." You have all the tools in your brain right now. You can be whomever you chose to be today. You don't need to read another book on dieting. No more searching for the magic pill that will melt it all away. No more buying expensive gym equipment. You have everything you need right now, inside yourself. When you follow this principle, you will trust that your unconscious mind will guide you to find the tools and present to you everything you need.

Keep your eyes open and trust your unconscious mind to show you everything you know and trust that it will make sure that you get introduced to the right people, the right material, the right ideas. When you set your unconscious mind on a mission, it keeps working for you in the background as you continue to live your life. It makes sure that things happen well for you.

KEY CONCEPTS:

NEED

People have all the resources they need to succeed. You can stop looking for external solutions to your problems. It is all there waiting for you inside.

CHAPTER 18

NORM

EACH PERSON HAS HIS OR HER OWN UNIQUE MODEL OF REALITY

Norm. You have your own way of establishing your norm. Your world is quite different than everybody else's. Even if the Internet and its tools allow us now to see maps in real time, with landscapes and buildings, it is never like being there for real and if we are there for real, we never really get the full extent and all the details of the location where we are. Even if you can make a mental picture of an apple, there is no apple in your head, it is not a real apple, it is only a picture of an apple. There is so much information thrown at us every second that we filter it and remember only a portion and make an idea for ourselves of what this place looks like. The map is not the territory. The way we represent the world refers to reality. It isn't reality itself. We don't respond to reality. We respond to our internalized map of reality. Interpretations may or may not be accurate. Our understanding of the world is based on our own experience and how we represent it. Whatever we think is going on, it's just what we think of it, it is not the real thing. That is our interpretation of how we see things.

Here is an easy way to represent this concept. Pretend that someone who is afraid of snakes sees a snake on the garden path. Their heart starts to beat faster, they start to sweat, the adrenaline goes up, the fear grows and their inner-self goes mad. Now, just as they are about to run as fast as they can in the opposite direction, they realize that it's a garden hose and suddenly feel completely better. In their model of reality, because they are afraid of snakes, their reality created a series of behaviours and they acted as if it was true. Your unconscious mind doesn't know reality. It only knows what you make of it.

We are all different. Some of us think in visual images. Some like sounds and words. Some are primarily aware of body sensations. When we map our world, we delete and restore information we receive through our senses. Then, when something happens to us, we quickly classify the experience based on our pre-conceived idea on the subject. We distort everything to make it fit our reality. We tell ourselves a modified story of what happened. A story from which we have deleted, restored and generalized information.

Preconceived notions are the locks on the door to wisdom
Mary Browne

Let's say for example you have a belief that the whole world is against you. Whenever you see people that are there to help, you will delete them quickly and not pay attention to their offers to help you. You will distort people's comments to make them sound like they are out to get you, and you will generalize the one time that it happened, pretending that this is ALWAYS like this and make your belief true. We all have beliefs. The more we challenge them, the more we can see changes and transform our beliefs into more useful and resourceful ones.

Let's say you think you are fat. When someone gives you a compliment and tells you: "Wow, you look great in this top", you complete the sentence in your head with "Yeah, she probably thinks that I am fat and she is trying to make me feel better". You have ignored the compliment, you have distorted it to fit your "fat-reality" and you are now generalizing it and everything you hear is always about your weight.

In a seminar recently, I pointed at one of my participant's shirt - she was wearing a championship's slow-pitch jersey - and was about to ask, "Are you still playing slow-pitch?" and she interrupted my sentence. I only had time to say: "Are you still....." and she said: "Pregnant? No I am just fat." Interesting how her own model of reality made her think that I would even say something like that. I was just asking her if she still played baseball!

Now what if it did happen to you for real that someone once told you that you were fat. That memory might be quite distorted. Maybe they said it just like that, or maybe they said, you are not at your best in these pants and you took it like an abrupt *you're fat* comment. You only get affected if you believe that fits you. Change your belief and it won't affect you anymore. Instead, that kind of comment reinforces the belief and limits you. Then it is not long before all you can hear are comments about your weight even when they have nothing to do with it.

When we look at the same things with different perspective, the more detailed our map is, the more freedom and flexibility we get. We also have to make sure our map is up to date and do a reality check from time to time. Have you ever been caught by a GPS when it takes you somewhere not knowing about the new road that has been built? Then it goes "*Recalculating*" on you?

Sometimes we imagine constraints and barriers that do not exist. We try something that did not work before and keep doing the same thing. If nothing changes, nothing changes. There is a popular definition of insanity and it's to do the same thing over and over and expect different results. What that really means for me is that we keep trying to change our behaviours when what we need to change is our beliefs. Our future has not been read yet. Let's not let anyone, not even our own map, convinces us of the contrary. It is not about who is right and who is wrong and it is not about what is true either. A map helps us feel resourceful and makes us see things from a different perspective. What people say they do and think they do is often far from what they actually do.

> *Beliefs have the power to create and the power to destroy. Human beings have the awesome ability to take any experience of their lives and create a meaning that disempowers them or one that can literally save their lives.*
>
> Tony Robbins

If we are operating within our model of reality, then we are always right. Our mental map limits what we're capable of, more often than external reality limits us. If we have obstacles in our head, they are worse than the external reality. The chocolate cake doesn't walk out of the fridge and into your mouth. There's always going to be an excuse, and it's our brain and mental map that creates the excuse.

In your model of reality, whatever works for you will show up. Let's say you have never noticed the brands of cars that were driving by you every day on your way to work. All of a sudden, as you are shopping for a BMW X1, they start popping out everywhere. You start seeing them all the time, everywhere! Do you always happen to notice your own car - or similar - when you drive by your "twin"? Once well programmed, trust your own model of reality to tell you what to do with everything that you see and that is stored inside you. Put your model of reality to service and change that model of reality to better suit your desires. If you live in a model that says that you are thin and healthy, you will suddenly start noticing the opportunities to stay fit (instead of finding excuses). You will be attracted to the healthy items on the menu and not even notice that they were giving out free cake that day. Allow your unconscious mind to do the necessary tweaking that will serve you even better. In order to do that, we need to work with the neurological levels of the mind.

KEY CONCEPTS:

NORM

Each person has his or her own unique model of reality. Everything we do, think or feel is interpreted by our own way to see the world. As we understand how our behaviour is tinted by our model, we understand how changing the model at the base will be more effective than trying to change the behaviour itself.

CHAPTER 19

NEUROLOGICAL LEVELS

Neurological levels. Let's start by looking at these neurological levels of the brain. Where are the behaviours classified in our brain and where are the beliefs? How does that work?

Robert Dilts' Neurological Levels model helps individuals align their environment, behaviours, competencies, beliefs/values, identity and purpose, challenging them also to consider a higher purpose – whether work-based, family, social or spiritual in which they make a contribution outside the day to day demands of life.

In coaching, my job is to help the client identify where the problem resides so that we can fix it right there. For each area, I will give you some example of what I mean by fixing the problem where it belongs.

There are 5 areas of a person's self that lead to our life purpose:

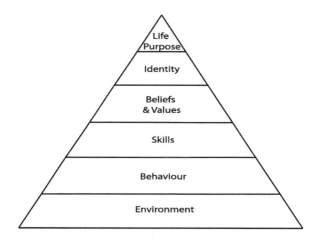

ENVIRONMENT

The environment is where we live, work, drive, play and exist. Our surroundings: the people and places where and with whom are interacting, and responding to, when we are engaged in a particular activity. It is at the base of who we are but it is not who we are. In the materialistic world we live in, a lot of people tend to identify themselves by the size of house they live in, the type of car they drive, the electronic devices they use or the brand of clothes they wear. But in fact, none of that "stuff" represents who we really are. It is just part of our environment.

As an example of looking into environment to fix a client's problem, you can refer to the lady I coached that was working in Saudi Arabia. She had an environment problem. She wanted to move to a different country and relocate her humanitarian work. At first, she thought that she needed to go back to school and work on her skills so that she could get a different kind of job, but when we turned into her values and beliefs, we found out that she was doing exactly the job she wanted. Her everyday life behaviours were great and she felt like she could be herself. The problem was her environment. She needed to do exactly the same thing, but in a different environment. She has now moved to Germany and is happily pursuing her career in the same field, in a totally new setting.

BEHAVIOUR

The behaviour is what we do (i.e.) salesperson, retiree, hairstylist, teacher. This could include, for example, what an observer would see or hear or feel when they are engaged in a particular activity. That includes interactions with your family, co-workers and friends. That also includes your activities like eating, exercising (or over-eating and lack of exercising). This is the level where most diets and activity plans are directed in order to help your weight-loss

NATHALIE PLAMONDON-THOMAS

journey. Changing the behaviour might work if the actual reason for over-eating or making bad choices resides in the behavioural layer of your own self. However, most of the time, the problem is in the values or beliefs' layer and cannot be fixed at the behavioural level. If a problem resides in the identity or the belief system of a person, that is where the problem needs to be addressed. This explains why some of the past attempts to lose weight failed. It is because it was not addressed at the right level. If you believe you are fat - belief and values level - then exercising and eating well - both behaviours - will not fix the problem. You will keep self-sabotaging yourself until you correct the belief.

CAPABILITY AND SKILLS

Capability is our skill, what we're good at and whether or not we have innate capabilities and/or learned skills for dealing appropriately with an issue. We are not necessarily born with skills. We develop them as we age with our life experiences. When we use our skills and do what we are good at, we more likely feel in harmony with ourselves. When using our skills, we avoid that sense of wasting our talent. You have likely heard the saying: "Chose a job you love and you will never have to work a day in your life". In this context, it makes total sense. When we are good at something, we more likely love doing it. And we love doing more of it.

What are you really good at? What are the things that are very easy for you to do without even thinking about them? What made you decide to buy this book? It's awesome that you have it in your hands and you believe that there's something here that can help you. You gave yourself that motivation. You gave that to yourself because unconsciously, you knew you were ready for the next level. Our skills give us confidence and strength.

Write down things you are really good at, skills that you do effortlessly. The things that people say about: "I don't know how you do it! There is no way I could do this." That means that it is a skill. Everybody can brush their teeth, which is a behaviour, but not everybody can remember the words of all the songs they hear. That is a skill. Name some things you do well:

_____

_____

_____

I was coaching a female police officer. She wanted to change her unit and to move up to a different level in the police force. She had tried unsuccessfully. She had even moved to a new city in order to apply in a different township, thinking she might have a better chance. It turned out that she had a skills problem. She was trying to fix it by changing her environment - moving to a different city - when in fact, she needed to take a few courses in order to upgrade her skills. She was convinced that she was capable of doing it - she had the proper belief and values in order to achieve her goal so the problem was really a skill problem. Again, identifying where the problem resides is key to fixing it. She did take the up skill course and was able to apply for a higher ranking position within the same division. She is now managing the Evidence department and feels totally fulfilled by her work. She is loving her job again!

BELIEFS AND VALUES

Whether we believe something is possible or impossible, whether we believe it is necessary or unnecessary, whether or not we feel motivated about something is all driven by what is imprinted in our unconscious. This level is critical when I work with my clients. What they believe is true, in their own representational systems, is forming who they are. Beliefs are at the base of our habits (good or bad). They are the main focus in the NEW YOU section of the D.N.A. System. We need to change our old negative beliefs in order to replace them with beliefs that will serve us better.

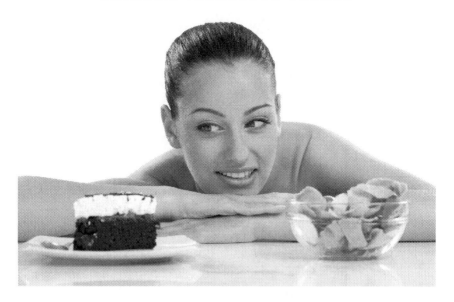

I have given you some examples where some clients had environment, behaviour, or skills problems. These three are not the most common. Most people's problems reside in the beliefs, values and identity levels. The closer to the base of the pyramid, the easier it is to fix. You run out of milk, you go buy some. The closer to the identity level at the top, the more you see it as a real problem. An easy example for this is when someone has a self-confidence problem (belief) and to give themself some more prestige and power, they buy themself an expensive sports car. The problem is in the belief level (self-confidence) and they are trying to fix it in the environment level (sports car). It can't work. Again, the problem needs to be addressed where it belongs.

Our beliefs and values are guiding all our actions. When they make us grow and give us fulfilling lives, we can thank them for making life easy for us. When, on the other hand, they make us see the world from a negative angle, we wish we could change them. The beliefs that are not serving us are called limiting beliefs.

Here are some limiting beliefs that we can address in the context of this book:

In this section, I am addressing the belief in itself. You will see how to change these limiting beliefs later on in the "NEGATIVE TO POSITIVE" section.

- LOSING WEIGHT IS HARD. Says who? What if you chose to believe that losing weight was easy? More likely, if you believe that losing weight is hard, then you are telling your brain and programming it to make it difficult for you. Every time you think about this statement, or every time you say it out loud, you are giving a reason for your brain to make it hard for you.

- DIETING IS TEMPORARY. Unfortunately, most people start a diet and give themselves a deadline. They say: "For the next month, I will not drink any wine, nor eat any cheese." But then, what happens in a month? When they start drinking wine and eating cheese again? Is the new state of mind supposed to be over? Were they conditioning themselves all along to only be able to avoid unwanted food for a certain period of time? Were they even programming their brain to crave it even more than ever at the end of the said time?

- WHEN YOU GO BACK TO EATING NORMAL STUFF, YOU GAIN THE WEIGHT ALL BACK, WITH INTEREST. This belief is not serving you either. The whole idea behind mind shifting is not to make you live on a lettuce and cucumber only diet for a short period of time and then gain it all back once you start having burgers and fries more often than you even used to before the diet. This belief should be transformed all along into a belief that you will not even go back to eating "normal stuff". What is "normal" anyways?

- MY FAMILY IS OVERWEIGHT. IT'S GENETIC. Really? Have you ever met someone skinny who has fat parents? If it is possible for one person, it is possible for you. The whole science of NLP is based on modelling. You can chose to model your parents or you can chose to model your healthy friends or anyone that feels comfortable with their weight.

- THAT IS MY PHYSIOLOGY; I AM DOOMED TO STAY THIS WAY. We all have a body-type of course. The skeleton of our body will more likely stay where it is. A 5 foot tall man cannot decide to become a 6 foot tall person by changing his belief. If you have wide shoulders and are tall, wearing size 10 shoes, you cannot dream to become a petite fragile lady wearing Cinderella's size 5. It won't happen. What can you dream then? You can visualize yourself being the best of you. Your own personal version of a perfectly healthy body.

- NO MATTER WHAT I DO, I CAN'T LOSE WEIGHT. Nothing ever worked? Ever? What would happen if you did? Have you ever thought that this belief, and its constant repetition in your head, might be the main reason that have kept you from losing weight all these years.

- I DON'T HAVE WILL POWER SO I CAN'T LOSE WEIGHT. How does not having will power cause you to choose to believe that you can't lose weight? Are these things even connected? Is will power not only an invention that we use as an excuse for our wrong-programming?

- I CANNOT LIVE WITHOUT CHOCOLATE. Okay, I tend to agree with this. That is totally true! Just kidding. What would happen if you did live without chocolate? How much chocolate do you really need? Is it a *need* or is it a *want*? And what makes you *want* this chocolate? When specifically do you decide that it is time for chocolate? What if we could re-wire your brain to have a different *want* at this exact moment?

- EATING WELL IS A LOT OF WORK. And being fat is not a lot of work? How about the hours you spent shopping for a simple outfit because nothing seems to fit right?

- EXERCISING IS HARD AND HURTS. Every type of exercise is hard? What if it could be fun? How would that be like if you enjoyed it? How about the first time you tried walking as an infant and fell. Thank goodness you kept trying and realized that walking is actually quite easy and doesn't hurt.

- I HAVE A SWEET TOOTH. Really? Your teeth are different than everybody else's? They affect your taste buds? Your taste buds have never changed before? How about the first time you tasted sushi or coffee? Did you like them at first taste? Did your taste buds adapt to them? What would happen if you stopped having a sweet tooth?

- I LOVE FOOD TOO MUCH! What makes you chose to think that this is a problem? What if you could direct this love toward the right food?

If you believe any of this, then that's what will happen. Remember, whether you believe you can do it or not, you are right either way.

Believe you can and you're halfway there.

Theodore Roosevelt

IDENTITY

The identity is who we are. Our self-esteem, our sense of self and what we identify with. This can include identifying with our job, marriage, religion, etc. It can also include how we interpret events in terms of our own self-worth. What we think we deserve or not.

Have you ever heard the expression: I AM a morning person. This is a deep belief engraved right at the identity level. We are not born to be morning or evening people. We chose to be more effective in the morning or not because we think so and we make the call. Saying the words: "I AM" a morning person is a symbol of a belief that is deeply engraved. It is much different than saying: "I work well in the morning or I get up early" which are behavioural affirmations and not identity related.

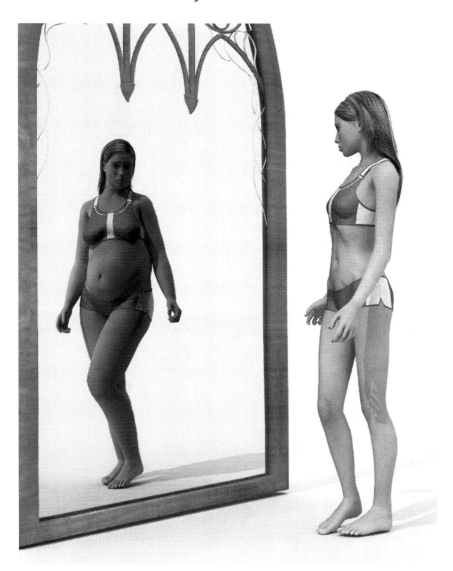

When we believe to be a person with big bones or a wide strong build or we say to ourselves: "I am a size 16", or "In my case, it is genetic, everyone in my family is big and have always been for generations" or "I am Indian and the sauces and the food are part of our culture, it is who I am" or "I am a foodie and I love food"

(identity level), buying an elliptical machine (environment level) or starting an exercise program (behaviour level) is not enough to fix the problem. Are you seeing the nuances now between all the levels? Please nod so that I know that you got it. Just kidding, I cannot see you, but I know you are nodding!

Understanding each level of our own self and identifying where the problems lay is a great step towards fixing it. When I hear people say: I am fat, the words I AM are very powerful, that means that they don't only think of themselves as having a big belly or a big butt, they say I AM, which refers to their identity level.

When we implement change, the higher we go on the neurological pyramid, the deeper we need to dig in order to make the change. By changing cars or clothes, we are only changing an environmental aspect of our life. But by changing who we are, we lose, in some aspect, a portion of who we are.

Most people are really reticent to change as nobody wants to lose their own self. Who are they going to be if they cannot be who they thought they were all their life? That is when re-writing our software and deciding what and who we want to be is an empowering tool that allows us to let go of our old self and embrace our new identity. My Indian friend in Calgary has changed her conception of her identity and detached it from the food she was eating. In changing her diet, she has lost tremendous amount of weight. I asked her if she felt like she was less Indian now? She responded: "I am more than ever, and now a gorgeous and self-confident one!"

"All that we are is the result of what we have thought."
Buddha

LIFE PURPOSE

When all the layers of the pyramid are aligned and we live in a wanted environment, doing what we are good at and following our beliefs and values, then we can really feel like we are being who we are and living our real life purpose. Our life purpose is the reason why we were put on this earth. Who else are we serving? What is beyond ourselves? Who else are you serving with your life? What cause is close to your heart?

We can use the model to recognise how the various levels interact and how they are related. And it provides a means of recognising at which level a problem is occurring and recognising the most appropriate level at which to target the solution.

Here is one last example: I was coaching a businessman client who wanted to advance his career. One of his fundamental values is family. One of his complaints about work is that he has to work late. And he's annoyed that he misses out on seeing his kids. He also holds a competitive trait as a fundamental value. So both of these values had to be addressed. He is a businessperson and he is a father. A happy person is a person who does what their highest purpose in life is and uses their skills following their beliefs and values. It's important to understand where you are at and how to tweak your life to work with each of these things. We realized that his family was more important to him than his career. So unconsciously, he was 'sabotaging' his possibilities of advancing in the company because he knew (again unconsciously) that it would mean seeing less of his kids. We then figured how to consciously satisfy his competitive desires while remaining on track with his family values. He is now happier at work where he has set some boundaries and works hard while he is there but is not staying after hours every day to satisfy his competitive nature. Instead, he has signed up for a hockey team and plays with friends twice a week, which satisfy his competitive thirst and also keeps him fit.

KEY CONCEPTS:

NEUROLOGICAL LEVELS

Our brain classifies information into different levels in the brain. Environment. Behaviours. Skill. Beliefs and Values. Identity. Life Purpose.

We need to identify where the problems are and fix them where they originate.

Beliefs and Values along with Identity are the main areas where the deeper problems reside.

Nutrition and Exercise are behaviours. If the unsuccessful weight loss is due to a belief problem, changing a behaviour will not fix it.

CHAPTER 20

NEGATIVE TO POSITIVE

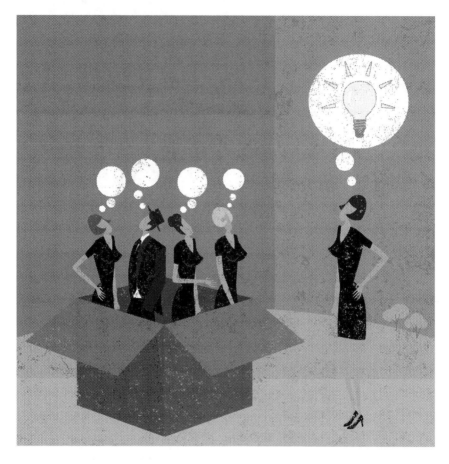

N egative to Positive. We have learned in the neurologic levels section how the beliefs and values are crucial and how they can affect our behaviours. The problem occurs when these beliefs are negative. We call them limiting beliefs.

The exercises below are different processes that will open up the boundaries of your unconscious limits. When you are in a problem box, sometimes you don't even realize it. These exercises will create windows and open up the walls so that you can see outside the box. The realizations that will occur as your walls go down will generate the light bulbs in your head in order for you to get the motivation you need to let go of the old beliefs. It will make you recognize that these beliefs that you thought were part of your life, are only true in your head and are not serving you. Therefore, they must go.

We will learn in this section how to turn them from negative to positive using our linguistic.

The power of words is very strong. You can actually breakdown any problem linguistically. As you will learn how your words impact your behaviours, you will start noticing your thoughts and you will be able to mentally hit the Cancel button whenever you get a negative thought. You will catch yourself having a negative thought and replace it with a good thought.

It starts right now with the most frequently asked question. When people ask you: "How are you doing?" create your own response. Use your words to create your situation. Pretend. Watch your language. Our words become our thoughts and our thoughts become our beliefs and our beliefs become who we are. Think about it wisely next time you are about to respond: "I'm okay, how are you?" Okay? That's it? That is all you aspire? You just told your brain that you want to be only *okay*. Not more. What will happen if you take this opportunity and every time someone asks you how you're doing, you can say: "I'm great", "I'm awesome", and "I'm majestic". You might as well program your brain to be amazing!

How about the anticipation of a feeling? Something that is not happening yet but that we plan ahead to feel bad. I once asked someone the million dollar question: How are you? She said: "I am tired! Well, I am not tired now but I will be by the end of the day. I have so much to do and I have to pick up the kids after work and bring one to soccer, one to guitar lessons and I will probably get stuck in traffic and get pissed off." So I asked: "Are you tired now?" She said: "No, not yet." "Are you in traffic now?" I asked. She said: "No not yet." So, I said: "Why are you already programming yourself to be tired? Why aren't you saying instead: "I will feel so great tonight because I will have accomplished a lot in my day. I will take advantage of the traffic to catch up on my audio book that I have been listening to. It will be awesome! Also, while my son is at soccer, I will drop my daughter to guitar and take 20 minutes to go for a short run to energize myself before I go pick them up again at the end of their sessions."

Do you have a global positioning system? A GPS? When you get off track and decide to turn when it is not time, what does the GPS say? Recalculating! So that is what I would like you to do every time you get off track. When you hear yourself say, "Chips are my downfall", quickly hear yourself say, "Oh, wait, what did I just think? *Recalculating.* Chips used to be my downfall but now I am easily choosing healthy food when I crave something salty and if I want to nibble on something, I am really into the snap peas - they are crunchy and I really love them."

Here is your chance to start to *Recalculate* more of your thoughts. The next series of questions will bring more digging to find out what has been keeping you from reaching your goals. What belief do you hold that could be transformed to serve you better? You know the nasty voice you hear in your head? You know exactly what I am talking about.

If you misfile, you can re-file. Is it your belief that when you lose weight you will gain it back? Is it your belief that losing weight is hard? It could just as easily be easy. You have to believe that it's easy and that it will work.

How do you feel about losing weight? What is your belief about weight loss? Do you believe you'll ever be your ideal healthy weight? You can choose to believe otherwise. We are the results of what we think and what we have been thinking our whole lives.

Ask yourself how does the idea of weight loss makes you feel? The universe wants to make you right. Everything that you create will make you right. So be really careful what you want to be right about.

Now that you know that something has been misfiled, you can re-file it again. We can choose what we do and what we think. We can make it fabulous. Listen to your own internal dialogue and listen to other people because that tells you about your own beliefs.

How do you feel about weight loss?

_____

_____

What is your belief about weight loss? Does it have to be hard?

_____

_____

How can you change this belief?

_____

_____

Do you believe you'll ever be your ideal healthy weight?

_____

_____

How can you change this belief?

_____

_____

How would you rather feel and believe about weight loss?

_____

_____

Now you know that you have a choice. Continue to believe this or change the way you see the whole thing. Take a moment to re-write these beliefs, choosing to turn them into something that will serve you better.

When we have a problem, the problem doesn't matter; the main problem is that we spend so much time on it that if we do get rid of it, we start filling up our head with negative thoughts. We focus on the wrong thing. Our brain has to say no to something, so we visualize the wrong thing and then negate it. At this point, once we have visualized the wrong behaviour and then have to reverse it, we are already heading in the wrong direction. Remember Mickey Mouse in his yellow tuxedo?

Disappointment requires lots of planning. If we begin to look at things as if they are difficult, they will be. If we study what makes things impossible, we will find out. We plan way in advance to be disappointed. If we think something will be hard and strenuous, it will be. It is setting us up for failure. If we are doing something and it is not working, there has got to be an easier way. We have got to do something else. And the first thing we have to do is to change our internal state. It begins with our thoughts, and thoughts become actions and actions become habits and habits become beliefs and beliefs become who we truly are.

There are many ways to enhance your language.

Use your senses when you re-phrase them. Make it happen in your head with visual, auditory and feelings. What's going to happen when you start believing these things? You're going to see yourself eating the vegetables. Visualize yourself reading a book of healthy recipes. Hear yourself order healthy choices at a restaurant. Feel how it feels to be walking with friends. Visualize yourself joining a fitness class with friends. What are the next steps? How are you going to feel when you're at work, taking a pass on the office doughnuts? How are you going to feel when you can say "I eat well". You need to build up unconditional compliments for yourself.

You know all the negative feelings that come with the limiting belief: "I can never resist ordering a burger in restaurants." What do you see in your head right now? What is the old image that you see when you hear yourself saying this limiting belief? Are you in a pub ordering? Is it noisy in there? What do you hear? What are you saying to the waitress? How do you feel? Are you really craving the sweet potato fries? Do you feel guilty already?

By changing the statement, you want to also change the image that is triggered in your head. So now, let's take the same limiting belief: "I can never resist ordering a burger in restaurants". Now re-write it and change it to: "I always choose the healthiest thing on the menu." Now make a mental picture of what it will look like. What is the ambiance in the restaurant? What do you hear yourself say to the waitress now? How do you feel? Do you feel amazing ordering your salad? See yourself getting excited and devouring this delicious healthy choice. Feel proud. Add all the senses that you need to make this statement real and compelling.

Avoid the "do not". Stop "trying" and just do. Don't use "if", use "when": "When I get to the gym...", instead of "if I get to the gym". Instead of saying: "I'm going to try and eat small healthy meals today", say "I am eating small healthy meals today." Not "I will", nor "I'm going to". You have to say: "I am". Use the present tense.

- I am in my perfect body.
- When I get to the gym today...
- It's easy to lose weight.
- I love vegetables.
- I crave fresh mangoes.
- I stay away from chocolate cake very easily.
- My butt is getting smaller.
- I am a manager of my body.
- I am losing weight.
- I am reaching my optimal weight.

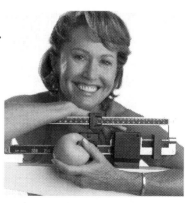

- I am releasing unwanted weight.
- I am increasing strength.
- I am enhancing my lean body mass.
- I am achieving my goal.

Here are the limiting beliefs that we have identified in the Neurological Section of this book. Let's have a second look at them and see how we can re-phrase them.

- Losing weight is hard = **Losing weight is easy.** This time it will be different. I know I used to think that way and that is the reason why I thought it was hard because I had chosen to think it was. Now that I am seeing it as easy, I will lose weight easily.

- Dieting is temporary = **My new body is permanent.** I am choosing a healthy lifestyle for good. I used to be on these diets and I now know that these temporary solutions are just that, temporary. I am now starting a new life and loving it.

- When you go back to eating normal stuff, you gain the weight all back, with interest = **I will keep my body healthy and thin because the changes that I am making now are permanent.** I am only attracted to healthy food now and my old "normal stuff" has totally changed.

- My family is overweight. It's genetic = **I used to have many excuses that were not serving me, and now I realize that I can manage my own body and I can be at my best, independently of any genetic factor.** I now choose to believe that I can be like lots of other healthy and fit individuals that also have overweight people in their family. Even if I have some obesity genes in my body, I also have a lot more healthy genes that can easily outnumber the unwanted ones. So I now focus on the good ones!

- That is physiology; I am doomed to stay this way = **Considering my physiology, I am at the best I can be.** I keep aiming at the best version of myself. I love my body-type and my bone structure and I feel amazing in my skin!

- No matter what I do, I can't lose weight. = **I can lose weight easily and permanently.** I have lots of different options to choose from as everything always works well. My day-to-day and my whole lifestyle is designed to bring me to a perfect weight and maintain it.

- I don't have will power so I can't lose weight. I used to think that will power had something to do with losing weight. **I can lose weight easily because I have a well-programmed brain.** My conditioning keeps steering me in the right direction.

- I cannot live without chocolate. = **I can easily pass on chocolate.** I used to like it and somehow, now, I am very happy without it. I crave sweet mangoes and peaches instead.

- Eating well is a lot of work. = **I have a great habit of eating well and it is easy and simple.** It is now part of my life and I have found great quick healthy ideas that work well for my lifestyle.

- Exercising is hard and hurts. = **I have found the perfect fitness routine for me and I enjoy my workouts very much.** I have lots of variety of exercise and I get a lot of satisfaction when I push myself. I am driven by the great results I get and I am stunned at how much fitter I am getting and how easy and natural it has become compared to when I first started.

- I have a sweet tooth. = **My taste buds are geared towards healthy food.** It is amazing how one's food preferences can change easily. I used to like sweet things and I now avoid them very easily.

- I love food too much! = **I love healthy food!** I use my natural foodie skills to discover and learn constantly about the new healthy trends and I am very good at transforming some of my old favourites into succulent healthy versions. I eat slowly and savour my food as I love it!

It's your turn now. You have read lots of examples and you are ready. List the things that you hear yourself say that are self-limiting, such as "losing weight is hard", "I will probably gain it back", "I have a big butt". I don't know what to eat", "I'm always tired", "I have food cravings all the time".

1. _____

2. _____

3. _____

4. _____

5. _____

6. _____

7. _____

8. _____

9. _____

10. _____

Use your linguistic (words) to re-phrase your limiting beliefs. Re-write them in a way that they can serve you. What should you chose to believe instead? How can you rephrase these to motivate yourself?

In order to help you with this exercise, here are some questions you can ask yourself in order to lower the intensity of the problems.

How? What? When? Where? And who specifically? (Do not ask why)

Says who?

According to whom?

Everybody?

Always?

Never?

Nobody? Nothing?

All? No one?

Compared to whom?

Compared to what?

How do you know? What stops you?

What would happen if you could?

What would happen if you did?

What would happen if you didn't?

So go ahead. Turn the negative into positive.

1. _____

2. _____

3. _____

4. _____

5. _____

6. _____

7. _____

8. _____

9. _____

10. _____

Once you have written them, repeat them as often as you can until they start becoming a part of you. These new beliefs are to be carried with your well-formed outcome. There are only ten here. You will want to pay real close attention to your thoughts and soon, you will be amazed at how easy it is to turn a limiting belief into a positive statement that will serve you. You will become a professional beliefs transformer. Watch your life go from a negative to a positive trend.

KEY CONCEPTS:

NEGATIVE TO POSITIVE

Our lack of success may have led us to create some limiting beliefs regarding weight loss.

As these beliefs dictate the way we act, we might as well change them in order for these beliefs to support our desires as opposed to stand in the way of realizing what we aim for.

You can start changing a belief by linguistically re-phrasing it.

CHAPTER 21

NEURO PATHWAYS

euro pathways. As you continue to use your linguistic to change your thoughts, you will be creating new neuro pathways inside your brain. That is how habits are created and formed.

The pathways along which information travels through the neurons (nerve cells) of the brain can be compared with the paths through a forest. As people keep taking the same route through a forest, they wear out a path in it. And the more people who take this path, the more deeply it is worn and the easier it becomes to follow. The same goes for our memories: the more we review them in our mind, the more deeply they are etched in our neural pathways.

Here is a quick exercise that will make you experience a different route for a neuro pathway that you have built throughout the years. If you're right-handed, try to write your name with the left hand, and vice versa. It's a very interesting exercise. We know how to write it and yet we can't do it very well with our left hand... but we could if we really had to. Create a new neural pathway to write it with your left hand. It's not that easy but you can do it.

- Write your name with your left hand - or reverse if you are a left-handed person:

How did it go? It is amazing how we can learn whatever we want. You can re-teach your brain to do things differently. Just practice. Repetition. Repetition. Repetition.

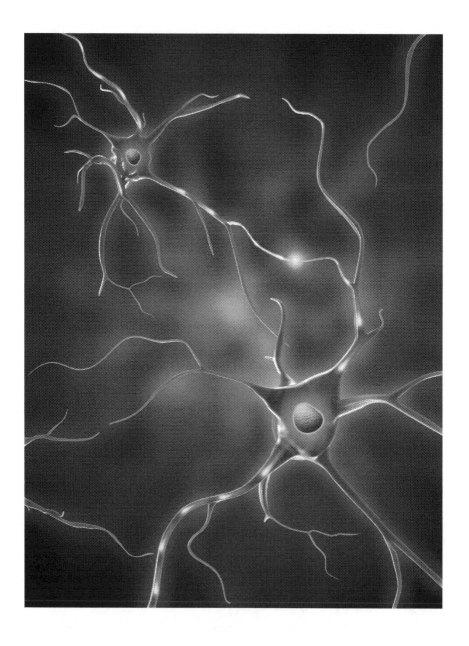

Success starts by expecting that you will be very successful at this. Your chances of losing weight and finally keep it off rely on what you expect to happen. Let me introduce you the notion of the placebo effect.

There has been diverse research conducted in Finland, Texas and Canada[8] on knee surgery. They had two groups of people who had knee problems. For the first group, they performed the actual surgery on the patient and fixed the knee. For the second group, they didn't perform the corrective surgery but the patient did receive a surgical scar. They did not tell the second group of patients that they were not receiving the surgery. They thought that they had been fixed. Both groups reported less pain and more mobility with their knee, regardless of whether or not they actually had the surgery.

This is a demonstration of the placebo effect. Medicine describes the placebo effect as a positive change in health that is not attributed to the treatment. That change can be from spontaneous improvement, misdiagnosis, classic conditioning or subject expectancy. The power of expectancy is a favorable response to a medical intervention that doesn't have a direct physiological effect (i.e. a pill, a procedure, a counseling session).[9]

It sounds very easy doesn't it? Well it is that simple! None of these patients had received extensive training in how to re-program their brain and how to create new neuro-pathways when it comes to the pain. But they were told to expect a different sensation when faced with the movement that used to cause them pain.

Let's take the example of a knee injury. Your brain has a blueprint of yourself in perfect condition. When you walk and everything is working normally, you don't feel any pain. So for your brain, the

---

[8] http://articles.mercola.com/sites/articles/archive/2014/02/07/arthroscopic-knee-surgery.aspx
[9] http://www.health.harvard.edu/mind-and-mood/putting-the-placebo-effect-to-work

action of walking equals no pain. One day, you hurt your knee. The brain creates a new neuro-pathway and it associates the action of walking to pain. So now, for your brain, walking equals pain. A new neuro-pathway has been formed. By repeating to your brain that your knee hurts, you are strengthening the belief and reinforcing the brain's new pathway. You are almost getting used to the pain. The longer it lasts, the more you expect it and the longer it takes to heal. By expecting to heal fast and doing something about the pain, we influence our brain to believe that it will get better. We let the brain know that the new neuro-pathway is only temporary and we actively ask for the old pathway to come back. We ask our unconscious to bring us back to the perfect blueprint of ourselves.

How many times did I hear in my classes someone say: "I cannot do that move because I have a knee injury (....)" and I wish the sentence would end there, but normally, it continues like this: "(...) and it has been years and I have learned to live with it. I have bad knees!!" So, they gave up! The new neuro-pathway has won over the old one. The person doesn't even remember how it feels to not have sore knees.

The activities you have performed so far and the ones coming up later in this book are all contributing to re-create healthy neuro-pathways. The best way to heal yourself or, going back to the subject of this book, to succeed in your weight-loss efforts, is to *expect* that it will work. Use the placebo effect to your advantage and tell yourself that you will be successful. Whether you THINK it is doable or not.... You are right either way. So start thinking that it is doable to ALWAYS make great choices.

We all create new neuro-pathways all the time (without knowing it). Every time we chose a new habit and stick with it for a while (moving from conscious incompetence to unconscious competence), a new neuro-pathway gets created.

Perhaps you have tried every diet on the planet; you might even have lost weight, a lot of weight, and if you are like most people, you have probably put it all back on again. Why? It is because you THINK of it as a diet. You think of it as TEMPORARY. You THINK it's impossible, and so, before you know it, and so that you don't starve, you find yourself back with your old poor eating habits, because they are familiar and comfortable.

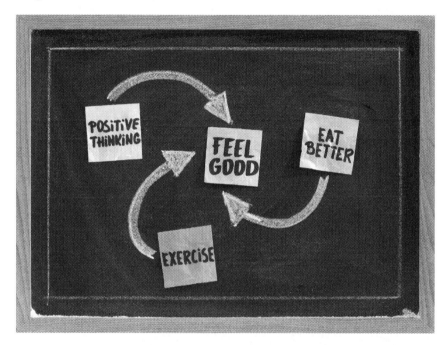

None of your patterns happened overnight. If you take sugar in your coffee, leave it out for about two months and you'll create a new neural pathway and you'll be used to your coffee without sugar. Habit is the key word. We want our health to be a habit, and not a diet. We see diets as temporary, and we want something that will last, that becomes a new behaviour, without effort.

At first we have to pretend until it becomes a habit, which can happen in 66 days. Pretend that you want the salad instead of the pasta. Pretend that you like vegetables until you actually do like them. Pretend that you like water instead of cola. You're pretending that you don't want or like the chocolate cake, until the new neural pathways are created. You choose, you decide. Change the way you think about food. Change the way you think about exercising. I love food. I love eating. I eat real food. I crave healthy things.

I used to love ice cream. That used to be my one "downfall" that I would allow myself once in a while. But I got rid of this *downfall* word a long time ago. Not only do I not crave ice cream anymore but, my mind is now so sure about the level of health that I want to reach, that my brain found a new way for me to avoid it. It made me not able to eat the ice cream because my teeth became sensitive to the cold. So now, I can't even eat it even if I wanted to.

I have to say that sometimes, in the summer, on the beach, I do go for a nice scoop of gelato. My teeth get sensitive and don't really like it. It makes me not want to repeat it anytime soon and I quickly forget about the fact that I just had ice cream. No guilt nor overthinking or analysing what impact this scoop of ice cream will have on me. I don't tell myself: "well, that will make me fat" or: "I will more likely gain weight with that" or, "well, I just screwed up my diet, I might as well have fish and chips tonight and a piece of chocolate cake... my day has already been ruined right?" Just forget about the ice cream and the fact that it ever happened. I know deep down (as I keep programming myself this way), that I will get back to my regular habit of eating clean and that my week will more likely present me with a few extra workout opportunities for this scoop of ice cream to be gone in no time. I know that I can get back easily to my blueprint of me, feeling great in my body. So there you have it. If you ask me: "Do you ever eat "bad" food?" I say "Yes, with pleasure." Often? "No. I don't crave them, they don't appeal to me but once in a while I do and I love every bite!"

Think about someone you know who is allergic to a certain food, that makes him or her sick. Do they have to use the so-called willpower in order to avoid the food? No. They are conditioned to easily avoid it because it makes them sick. What if you saw these devil foods for what they really are? Making you fat, bloated and sick! Could you avoid them too? The same way allergic people are avoiding the food that makes them ill? What is different about the way they think about these specific foods? You are starting to understand how this works, right?

You want to re-write your life. Create a new life, slowly, creating new healthy habits, rather than going on yet another 'quick fix diet'. How will you do it differently next time?

KEY CONCEPTS:

NEURO PATHWAYS

Our brain executes commands as it is told how to respond and reproduces the same response.

We get what we expect will happen.

Our life experiences create automatic responses in our head.

These automatic responses become habits.

CHAPTER 22

NEGATIVE NEURO PATHWAYS

Negative neuro pathways. What happens when you try a new diet and it doesn't work? It makes you feel bad. You think: "Oh, I was doing so well, I lost that weight and now I've gained it back." You feel like a failure. You feel bad and you resent the process. Everyone is telling you "eat well and exercise". If it's that easy, then why aren't we all thin? After all these failed trials at it, you want to shake them and say: "NO!!! It's NOT easy! It's actually really hard!!!"

All these years, you have been putting your money, time and energy into the exterior body of your car. You have put on shiny paint, safe tires, performance gasoline in the gas tank, etc. But if the car computer system is not taken care of as well, even the prettiest car will not perform. Similarly, you have been told for so many years that all you need to do is to exercise and follow a great diet. Today, you are learning the key component to your journey ... YOUR navigation system: YOUR BRAIN.

The reason why you may feel this way about healthy food and exercise is because you have some negative neuro pathways that have been formed around these subjects. What happens when we give up on the diet or don't make it into the gym? We probably blame ourselves and it makes us feel bad!!!

Instead of making us feel great, our nutrition and exercise make us feel crappy and discouraged. So we start to resent it and when we hear these words: Nutrition.... Exercise.... we remember how crappy we felt last time we tried.... And we are reminded of failure every time.... This turns into a barrier to our success and we keep the weight on. Do you relate to this? It's no wonder you keep giving up! Your mind is working against you.

You are now learning how to do it naturally and effortlessly and you will actually want to do it. What you have started with the exercises of this book is to re-create new neuro pathways for your brain. Now when hearing exercise and healthy food, you will start to light up and smile.

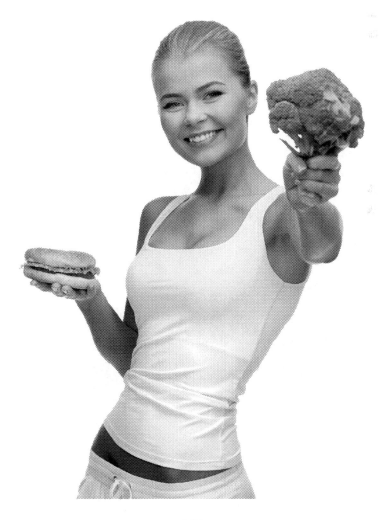

The pathway for successful nutrition and exercise had not been created yet. You are just starting and you are creating a new pathway for nutrition and health. Just like the exercise we did at the beginning of this section. Writing with our usual hand is easy and natural, whereas writing with the other hand requires the creation of a new neural pathway. As you would see if you were to practice the handwriting, creating new neural pathways can be done and it doesn't take that long. What if making good choices could be as natural as writing with your predominant hand? You can learn how to make the broccoli win over the burger every time!

In the ACTUALIZE section of this book, I will introduce a few more techniques to program your brain. They will help you get confidence, which, will, in turn, contribute to re-writing new neuro pathways that will make new habits easier to settle in your new life. For now, let's do a bit of cleaning. We have identified your limiting beliefs. We have re-phrased them. Even if you have some new cupboards to replace the old ones, it doesn't mean that there is room in your kitchen to keep them all - old and new ones. We need to remove the unwanted limiting beliefs and create more space for the new beliefs, elaborated above, to take roots.

KEY CONCEPTS:

NEGATIV NEURO PATHWAYS

The reason why we have not been successful in the past is because our brain created a habit of responding negatively to our weight-loss efforts.

By changing our limiting beliefs into positive beliefs, we are starting the process towards creating positive automatic responses.

CHAPTER 23

NEMESIS

Nemesis. The following exercise will teach you how to identify what you used to perceive as your limitations, your boundaries. See that as your personal nemesis. You have ideas about your weaknesses and your potential. Sometimes, you see your identity as set in stone and can't see the possibilities open to you. You will discover that you can be whatever you want to be. This exercise will help you shake the box so that you can get out of it. It will soften your limits and help you see yourself from your core, from within as opposed to see yourself from the outside, looking at your limitations.

Pretend that there are 6 squares on the floor. You will visualize the grid below as if it was on your floor and will physically step inside each square and answer the questions and do the mental work describe below. This grid is your identity matrix. It is your own self-concept.

3. LIMITATION	2. POTENTIAL	1. CORE
4. BOUNDARY	5. WEAKNESS	6. SHADOW

It is important that you physically stand up and move from one square to the other. When it comes to your mind, all the details count. You want to allow your unconscious mind to really distinguish each of these states and by physically moving from one space to the other, you will let it know that each concept is different from one another.

1. As you stand in the first square of the matrix, ask yourself the following question:

What do you believe you are and will always be? Something you are, at your core, you are happy to be that way, as you want to be like that, and you know in your core that you will always be it. What are you proud and content to be?

What symbol or picture can you make of this? What visually comes up to your head?

Write down your word (quality, state) in the first CORE square and draw or write down the symbol.

2. Move to the second square and ask yourself the following question:

What is something you want to be and believe you could become? Something you are hoping to become. Something you are excited about becoming. Visualise a symbol for it and write down your answer along with the symbol in the POTENTIAL square.

3. Move the third square and ask yourself the following question:

What is something you want to be but believe you are not? Something you see as your limit? You would like to be that way but you feel trapped and frustrated as you don't seem to be able to be it. What symbol can you think of for this? Record your answers in the LIMITATION square.

4. Move to the fourth square and ask yourself the following question:

What is something you don't want to be and never will be? You don't want to be that way and you feel very strongly about never becoming that way either. What is off limits? What is your boundary? You don't ever want to be that way. What does that look like? Give this a symbol and record your results in the BOUNDARY square.

5. Move to the fifth square and ask yourself the following question:

What is something you don't want to be but believe you could become? What is your weakness or your defect? Are you afraid you might become this? This may cause you anxiety as you don't want to be that way and you may become it. What symbol can you attribute to this? Record your answers in the WEAKNESS square.

6. Move to the sixth square of the matrix and ask yourself:

What is something you don't want to be but you are afraid you are? This is your shadow, something you feel guilty of or ashamed of. What visual can you connect to this? Record your answers in the SHADOW square.

Here is an example of a completed Matrix:

3. LIMITATION	2. POTENTIAL	1. CORE
I want to be and believe I am not: *Eating well* It looks like: *a burger*	I want to be and could become: *Active* it looks like: *a lady running*	I am and will always be: *Honest* it looks like: *a handshake*
4. BOUNDARY	5. WEAKNESS	6. SHADOW
I don't want to be and will never be: *looking like a toothpick* it looks like: *a toothpick*	I don't want to but I could become: *Sick from being overweight* It looks like: *a hospital*	I don't want to but I am afraid I am: *Lazy* it looks like: *a couch*

To continue the exercise, I will use the example above to make it easier for you to follow.

7. Now go back in square one and fully immerse yourself in your core. Visualize that handshake and feel that your core value of honesty is shining from the inside. Pump your chest up, stand tall and roll your shoulders back. Anchor that sense of honesty as your core and fully identify yourself with it.

8. Now keep your feeling of honesty glowing inside yourself as you step into the second square. Carry with you the handshake and incorporate the symbol with the image of the lady running. What do they look like together, what new symbol do you make of it? Keep your sure state of mind coming from your core (honest) and immerse yourself with the same assurance into being active. Imprint your core into the state of being active until you can feel about being active the same way you feel about being honest.

9. Now move to the third square and bring your integrated symbol with you along with your core and your potential. You are now fully honest and active. Imprint these feelings into the feeling of eating well. How can your honesty and you being active allow you to eat well and allow you to believe in eating well as much as you believe in being honest? Notice how your true core and potential can transform the symbol associated to your limitation. What does the symbol look like now? A handshake with a lady running and a new transformed symbol that represents eating well.

10. Step into the fourth square and bring your core and potential feelings with you along with your new symbol that includes eating well. Notice how your newly transformed self-concept helps you clarify your boundaries. What is different about the toothpick? How can your boundaries be wider? Or non-existent at all? What if your boundaries could go altogether?

11. Carry these new updates and clarifications into the fifth square along with your integrated symbol that includes the handshake, the lady running, the new symbol for eating well and the new symbol for the toothpick. Experience how your new learning can bring healing and transformation to your sense of weakness. How can

your core bring power to your sense of being active and eating well, and the fact that your boundaries are widening can help you avoid getting sick? Fully immerse yourself into your core and notice how your weakness changes in light of this new power from your core and potential. Does the symbol change?

12. Bring the integrated symbol into the sixth square and experience how this healing transformation from your core power can bring light into your shadow. What changes in the symbol of being lazy? How does that state change altogether? How does the symbol of the couch change now and integrate with the handshake, the lady running and the transformed symbols for eating well, released boundaries and new symbol for the hospital?

13. Return to the space of your core and fully integrate all your discoveries and transformation you have gained from each steps of the matrix. How do you feel now? What have you learned?

More than likely, now you have a very different view of yourself. You have opened up the mental process and set up a path favourable to transformation. It is like you have just lifted the old counter top with a crow bar and now it will be much easier to remove it from the counter and get rid of it.

Negative limits, shadows, weaknesses, defects or boundaries have been loosened up and they are ready to leave your body.

KEY CONCEPTS:

NEMESIS

We all have qualities that we are proud of and that we stand behind. These are part of who we are. They constitute our core.

We can use that core certainty to make our potential come true and use their combined strength to clear up our limitations, expand our boundaries, reverse our weaknesses and get rid of our shadows.

CHAPTER 24

NEW YOU ACTIVITY

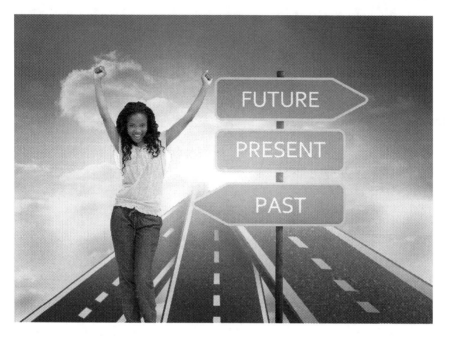

N ew You. This exercise is a very powerful technique that will help you release everything you are now ready to let go of and build a New You.

As mentioned in the Neuro Pathways section, you have been going through life and have had different experiences that made you create limiting beliefs about yourself. From these beliefs, you generated some unwanted behaviours that turned into bad habits. Here is the good news. All these experiences were far from negative. They were only feedback. They were only designed to make you learn something. When these experiences happened in your life, they were only there to get you to where you are today.

They happened to make you stronger and to make you grow. For every negative challenge that you experienced, a positive learning came with it. Unfortunately, this positive learning was attached to a negative feeling.

This exercise will help you detach the negative feeling from the positive learning so that you can let go of the negative feeling. We can make this negative feeling go away by telling the unconscious mind to acknowledge the positive learning from the challenge. Once this positive learning has been received, there is no need to keep the negative emotions anymore and your unconscious mind can release them.

In the middle of every difficulty lies opportunity.
Albert Einstein

I recommend that you read the exercise a few times so that you know exactly what to do once you close your eyes. Remember that your unconscious mind can process 2.3 million pieces of information every second. Your unconscious mind will know exactly what to do. Your logical mind might try to get in the way. Just ignore it. Trust that your powerful unconscious mind knows what to do. Take a moment to relax and get into a calm state so that you can give your unconscious mind a favourable environment to do its magic.

If you prefer to be guided by my voice and just sit back, you can purchase the recordings of these activities on my website www.dnalifecoaching.com Either way it works. Trust yourself.

Step one: How do you perceive time?

If I ask you to point to an area of the room where your present is and where your future is, where would you point? Is your past behind you and your future in front of you? Or is your past to your left and your future to your right? If you were to make a line from your past to your future, where would the line be? Would it be from back to front or from left to right? And where is the present? Is the line going through you and you stand in the present or is the line in front of you and you are looking at the line and can see the past, the present and the future? Are you standing in the line?

Step two: Noticing the present.

Physically stand up and allow your breathing to slow down and get into a state of comfort. Imagine time stretched out on the time line you have identified the above. Standing in the present, turn to look at your past and see what brought you to become who you are today. Have you constantly been gaining weight on a regular basis in the past? Have you tried to diet and failed? Have you been eating unhealthy food? Now turn facing the future, and take a few steps into your future to realize how it will feel in a year from now. If you don't change what you are doing right now, how will your future look? How will it feel ? Will you continue to gain weight if you don't make any changes to the way you eat, the way you exercise, and mostly, the way you think?

Step three: Negative emotion release

Now, step back into the present. Imagine yourself stepping up above your body and looking down at your time line. Look down at your past, present and future.

As you look at your past, you can see all those times when you had a bad experience. See every diet that did not work or every time that you gained the weight back. Every time you looked at yourself in the mirror with a sensation of failure. And as you look down, from up above, you can realize that each of these experiences was a training ground for your future. Notice the information that emerges from each of these experiences. Remember that your brain can process information very fast. Trust your unconscious mind to stop at every instance where it feels that you have had an experience from which some negative emotions stayed lingering. Ask your unconscious mind to take only the positive learning from that experience and to release the negative emotion. All you ever needed from this experience was that positive learning. And now, with that positive learning, the negative emotion will go away.

Let the new information float out as a radiant glow. Take that light with you and keep it available so you can use it in the future. Everything else - negative emotions and limiting beliefs - can exit your body and be released from your past. Come back from your past to the present, stopping at each event that has affected your weight loss journey, collecting the positive learning. Once back in the present, and once you have learned everything you need to acknowledge in order for the negative emotion to be released, open your eyes and feel how this new information will help you in the future. Notice how your future has now shifted and changed in light of that new learning.

Step four: Shift

Now close your eyes again and float way up in the air again. Look down and see how your past looks different now. Realize that all those experiences were just generative results and that you feel good about them now. Whatever troubled you has left and is getting further away by the second. As you feel good about your past, look down at your future and imagine the best kinds of feelings in it. Fill every future experience with the best state of mind. See your future looking better than ever.

Step five: Experience the future

From way above, looking down at yourself, go slowly back into your body and feel full of excitement, anticipating the most amazing future. See yourself in the best shape of your life. Experience the same you in a much healthier and happier body. Feel a life full of the most wonderful things, new people, new possibilities, new food, new activities, new habits!

Now physically step forward on your line towards the future. Notice how your whole future has now shifted and changed from what you experienced in the first part of the exercise. Feel how it feels to be lighter, to look exactly how you want to look, to feel how you want to feel, to hear others tell you how great you are and how radiant you look!

Step six: New You

You can now open your eyes and feel the new you transformed and ready for a compelling and exciting future. You won't stop having external pressure or challenges; you will simply be able to deal with them differently. In light of this new learning, you have now understood its purpose and how to release the negative emotions that accompany each learning experience. It doesn't mean that you will never have a negative emotion again; it means that if you go there, you won't stay there long. You now have the tools to get out of any problem box.

KEY CONCEPTS:

NEW YOU ACTIVITY

Although challenges are designed to teach us a lesson and make us grow, some experiences are causing us to create limiting beliefs. We can release them by acknowledging the positive learning that our life events brought to us.

CHAPTER 25

NEUTRALIZE THE PAST

N eutralize the past. The technique we just did was an exercise that will have taken care of all your limiting beliefs in general. Mostly, everything that has generated negative emotions has been lifted and is now exiting your body. It allowed you to shift your previous negative emotions into positive learning from your experiences.

Here is another technique that you can use in order to neutralize very specific incidents that you feel have caused you to be unsuccessful with your weight loss efforts. There might be some specific experiences that, once disconnected from your past, will allow you to better move on. In fact, sometimes we remember a negative experience because of how it made us feel. The experience in itself was not negative. Our response to it is what we remember. A state cannot be erased. It can only be replaced by something else, a more serving one.

In this exercise, you will remember an experience that you classified as negative and replace the feeling that this experience generates by positive feelings.

Step one: Getting into the replacement state

Now, think of a time when you were feeling on top of the world. Immerse yourself in this situation. Let that fantastic sensation grow, imagine it moving through your entire body. Take this feeling, give it the colour of your choice and imagine it springing through your past so that it covers every negative memory and every bad experience. Imagine soaking them with this really great feeling.

Step two: Identify the negative feeling you want to erase

Think about a part of your life when you felt stuck or blocked. Think of a moment that gives you bad feelings and limits your behaviour. Maybe an episode of binge eating or a time when someone you care about told you that you were fat.

Step three: White it out

Imagine watching the negative experience on a giant screen. Imagine a brightness button on the side of the screen. In one quick move, turn it all the way to the maximum brightness, until you white it out completely. One moment you see it and the next, it is completely whited out. Do it again. Imagine it and white it out really quickly. Repeat 2 or 3 times until it comes naturally.

Step four: Replace the state

Take the amazing feeling and as you imagine the difficult situation again, white out the negative feeling and spin this really good feeling in its place. Hear a confident voice say: "Never again!" Focus on the good feeling spinning fast in your body and notice the good feeling.

Step five: Shake your body and go back to a neutral state.

Step six: Verify the process

To verify that this new strategy works out automatically, think about the negative situation and see how you are feeling. Can you imagine feeling bad? How does that make your feel? Repeat the process until you feel great when you think about the situation.

You can also use the following similar exercise to achieve the same result with something you wish you were not doing anymore. This time, use a behaviour, instead of a feeling.

Step one: Getting into the replacement behaviour

Think of the last time you did something amazing like eating something healthy, getting to the gym and getting a good sweat, going to bed early or refusing dessert. Get into the pride generated by doing the right thing and how amazing it felt.

Step two: Identify the behaviour you want to erase.

Think of the last time you ate something you shouldn't have, or the last time you skipped your exercise and got lazy on the couch. Think of something that still bothers you. Think of something you don't want to think about anymore. Think of the visual representation, the image or movie you see in your mind's eye.

Step three: Make it disappear

Take a picture of the event and make it smaller. Move it far into the distance. Take the colour and the brightness out of it. If you hear voices and sounds of the scene, make them fade away. Make the picture so small that you have to squint to see it. Then make it even smaller. When it is the size of a breadcrumb, brush it away. Repeat the process three times.

Step four: Replace the state

As you make the image disappear, get into your replacement state and fully immerse yourself into the desired behaviour that you want instead.

Step five: Shake your body and go back to neutral.

Step six: Test

Think about the situation that used to generate a negative behaviour and notice if your first thought is not to do the positive behaviour instead. Repeat the process as many times as you need in order to make this happen naturally.

When you think about past bingeing experience or bad habits or things you shouldn't eat, make sure the image looks like a white Polaroid. Push it off into the distance.

KEY CONCEPTS:

NEUTRALIZE THE PAST

Experiences in life are neither positive nor negative. The way we respond to these experiences are making them good or bad. If a specific event causes us to have negative emotions, we can change the negative feeling by a more desired one.

Responses cannot be deleted; they can only be replaced. When a specific event causes us grief, we can change our response to the event by replacing it by a different behaviour.

CHAPTER 26

"A" FOR ACTUALIZE

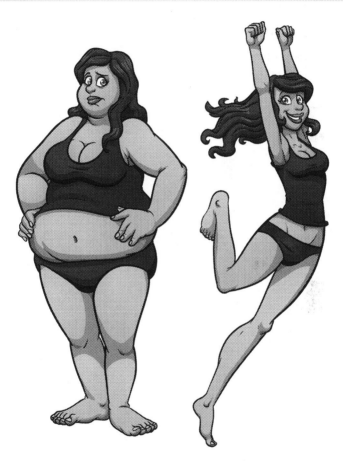

ctualize. Now that you have elicited your desires and created a New You, you are now ready to install the desires and program your brain with what you want.

The third component of the D.N.A. System is the ACTUALIZE section. It will teach you how to implement and cement your desires. You have chosen your new kitchen, you know exactly what you want, you have gotten rid of the old cupboards and now it is time to install the new ones and lay down the new marble counter top.

This section will not only allow you get a strong new foundation for your new thin life, it will also ensure you have the tools to get to the best you want to be and maintain your New You so that the weight doesn't come back.

You can use each of these processes separately. I suggest you do them one by one and take some time to implement each new achieved state before moving on to the next exercise.

KEY CONCEPTS:

ACTUALIZE

The third component of the D.N.A. System is the ACTUALIZE part. You will learn in this section how to implement and program your desires into your brain.

CHAPTER 27

AMPLIFY POSITIVE FEELINGS

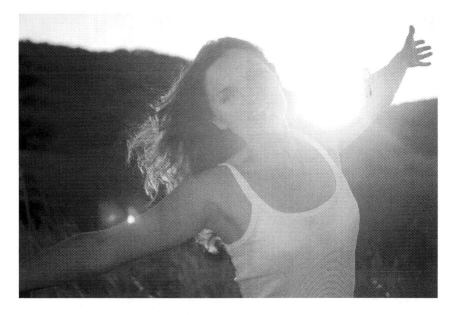

A mplify. People are drawn to your energy, to what you are and what you stand for. Not your skills or smartness or material possessions. They are drawn to the state you are in. The good news is that you can make yourself feel great by sending yourself nice messages on a regular basis. It is all about mental rehearsing. Remember things that make you feel good all the time. Expect to feel good all the time. Shift your belief that feeling good is only for special days. When you feel great, it is easy to exercise and to choose healthy food. Believe that life is meant to make you feel good all the time. Believe it so deeply that, unconsciously, your mind will do what is necessary to feel good.

This technique is designed to allow you to feel great and be your best whenever you want. Usually, diets start well; you are motivated and you are doing everything right. You are on a mission and you are getting results. You love it and it is even kind of easy. Then, somehow, it starts to plateau and you find your motivation lowering and somehow, all the great feelings you had are going down the drain and everything seems so much harder. How great would that be to be able to amplify your positive feelings so you can make them last? This is exactly what you will do with this exercise.

Step one: Identify a positive feeling to amplify

Close your eyes and think about one of the best feelings you have ever had in regards to your weight. You felt amazing. Maybe you were on a diet, maybe you were not. Either way, you had your Mojo going. See what you saw and hear what you heard when you felt that good feeling. As you do so, notice where this really amazing feeling comes from. Where in your body does it start? Where does it move? When you stop thinking about the feeling, where does it go? Notice the pattern of the feeling. Pull it back up and embrace it fully, then stop thinking about it and notice how it ends.

Step two: Amplification

Go back to that amazing feeling, and let it come up fully. Grasp it generously and just before it goes away, imagine pulling it out of your body and place it back where it begins, so that it moves in a circle. Spin it round and round and faster and faster. Notice that, as you spin it faster, the feeling gets stronger. Experience how much pleasure your body is truly capable of. Feel the exhilaration of this amazing state.

By doing so, you are reinforcing the neuro pathway that was created when experiencing this for the first time and you are amplifying the feeling and putting it at the top of the pile so that it is readily available for you whenever you feel that your motivation starts to deflate.

Being in a state of confidence helps in trusting your abilities to succeed. This time, whenever there are obstacles in your weight loss journey, you will be able to go right back into that resourceful state and find strength and energy to do whatever you need to do to make this work.

With amplified positive feelings, you don't have to know everything because it allows you to believe in your ability to learn and to adapt so you can continue to progress. Learn what needs to be learned and do what needs to be done. Will there be challenges? Maybe. You can power through anything. I know you already have a degree of excellence. You are here reading these pages aren't you? You have already committed. Now use this confidence to get to the next step and take action.

Repeat this exercise every day, and every time something great happens. Live it fully and amplify it. So that eventually, at the top of your pile, there will only be great amazing states ready to be experienced and re-loaded again to the surface.

KEY CONCEPTS:

AMPLIFY POSITIVE FEELINGS

You can mentally rehearse positive feelings and amplify them in order to have them accessible to you at any given time.

CHAPTER 28

ANCHORING

A nchoring. We just mentioned in Amplify Positive Feelings that the state you are in influences your results. Now we will learn how to actually recall one of these amplified feelings. It's just like pushing a "feel-good-button".

Here is an exercise to trigger a positive feeling with the skill of anchoring. You can use it whenever you are about to make a choice related to your weight-loss journey and, frankly, in any type of situation. We learned in chapter 11 to *Do it with your body and the mind will follow*, that the mind and body are connected. An emotional feeling can trigger a physical response and the reverse can also happen. A physical stimulus can trigger an emotional state.

Quality is not an act, it is a habit.

Aristotle

Step one: Recall the positive feeling to be anchored

Imagine a movie screen in front of you with a button control connected to what you see on the screen. Go back in your mind to a time, a specific time, when you had a really great experience. Feel the feelings that you felt back then. Perhaps you will imagine a scene when you were at your ideal weight. Or a memory of a time you were successful at skipping dessert or a time you know that you had lots of willpower. Feel free to use one of your previously amplified positive feelings.

Step one: Amplify the positive feeling to be anchored

Picture the image getting bigger and closer. Live it as the feeling increases. Be "associated", that is, be the main character, seeing the experience through your own eyes (as opposed to be a third person looking at yourself - dissociated). As this happens, imagine that the button control says 'awesome' and slowly imagine turning it up. To make it feel even more real, as the feeling intensifies, make the physical gesture with the button with your hand. As you turn it up, at the rate that fits the changes, allow that exhilarating memory to get closer, bigger and brighter. Add colour to it, make it shine, look at all the details. Hear a voice in your head that says: "I am awesome! This is amazing!"

Step two: Anchor

At this moment, when you are fully imprinted with the feeling, apply pressure to a part of your body which will become the kinesthetic anchor for this awesome state of mind. You can choose for the anchor to be a specific spot on your hand, on your knuckle, on the back of your neck, etc. Choose a specific spot that you can recall easily. Please avoid common anchors like pressing your hands together, which you do usually in other states (i.e. when you are nervous or when you are cold) because that could send wrong messages to your brain without you noticing. So choose something specific that will only be used to recall positive feelings.

Step three: Neutral

Enjoy this sensation for an instant or two, then release the anchor and let your body come back to a more neutral state.

Step four: Repeat

Repeat the process a few times. It is important to apply the anchor at the peak of the emotional state. It is really important that you do repeat the process at least three times in order to avoid sending mixed messages to your brain. So before going to step five, you must make sure that your brain knows exactly what to do when you press the anchor.

Step five: Test

To verify that the anchoring was successful, remember a moment when you were not at your best. Go there now and feel how it felt. In this negative state, the application of pressure on the anchor will reverse your state and make you feel great instead. Press the anchor as you say to yourself: "I am awesome!" You will find yourself going to a feeling as ecstatic as before.

You can chose anywhere on your body. I use a physical anchor on myself. I have a spot right behind my neck that I press firmly with three fingers every time I am in a great mood. When I finish a seminar that went really well, when I witness a client succeeding in something, at the end of a great fitness class where I was at my best, when something great happens to me or simply, when I feel like a million bucks! I have been anchoring these feelings right behind my neck for years. And now, whenever I need a boost, whenever some external pressure comes to me, I just press the back of my neck with my three fingers and my brain thinks that it needs to generate these exhilarating feelings, which works every time. I immediately get a rush of great warm sensations, which help me go through whatever is presenting itself to me at the time.

Remember to keep adding on to your anchor, anytime you experience a great feeling. First, amplify it and then anchor it. Keep stacking more and more so that you make your anchor solid and powerful.

SPACIAL ANCHORING

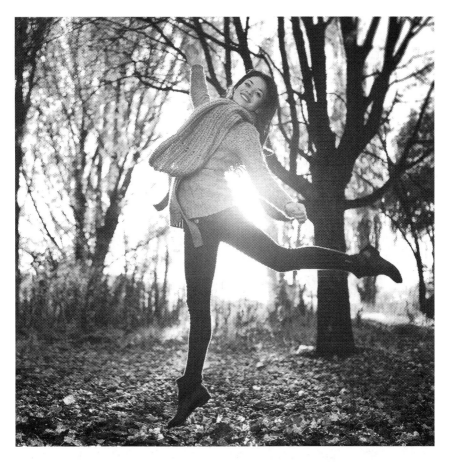

We have just learned physical anchoring. You can also use a space anchor. Here is the process that we call the Circle of Excellence.

Step one: Set up the space

Imagine a circle big enough so that you could easily step into it. Give it a colour and visualize it. Place it on the floor in front of you and stand just behind it.

Step two: Recall the positive feeling to be anchored

Think of a specific time when you were at your best or when you were easily able to perform the behaviour that you are trying to achieve. For example, if you are feeling lazy and don't feel like exercising, think of a time where you were going to gym regularly and effortlessly. Get into that specific feeling, the same way as above, being associated in the memory, seeing it through your own eyes and increasing the awesomeness of the event.

Step three: Anchor

When you are at the peak of the moment, step into the circle of excellence. Hold the feeling there for a moment until you feel that it starts fading away. When it does, leave the feeling in the circle as you step out.

Step four: Test

Test the circle of excellence. Get into a neutral feeling. Step into the circle of excellence. Notice if your mood changes and adopt the feelings that were left for you in your circle.

You can use the same circle for lots of situations or have different coloured circles that would match various desired states.

KEY CONCEPTS:

ANCHORING

You can store positive feelings in a physical or spatial anchor and recall them when you need them simply by triggering the anchor.

CHAPTER 29

ACT AND MERGE

A ct. In chapter 19 *NEUROLOGICAL LEVELS*, we learned that our identity is built with different layers. This exercise will place you in each neurological level in order for you to break down every level of yourself and assign a new reality to each part of you. You will assume a new environment, a new behaviour, new skills, news beliefs and values, new identity and new life purpose. You will use the neurologic levels to take action and figure out what you need in order to do or achieve your vision. Make a list of what you need to be or have in order for your desired outcome to actualize.

> *The ladder of success is best climbed by stepping on the rungs of opportunity.*
>
> *Any Rand*

Step one: Recall your desired outcome.

Go back to your desired outcome that we elicited in chapter 14 - *DARE*. Fully immerse yourself in the outcome. Go there in your mind as if it was happening right now.

Step two: Imagine someone to model.

Now as you are thinking about your outcome, step into the shoes of someone that has already achieved this outcome. Maybe it is you, ten years ago, when you had your Mojo. Maybe you know someone you can model. Maybe you want to model a healthy celebrity that seems to be how you want to be. You can also make a mental image of someone fictional that has achieved your desired outcome.

Step three: Environment

Imagine there are six squares on the floor in front on you, all in line with each other. The first square, the closest to you says: Environment. Step into this first square. Close your eyes and ask yourself what is the environment for the people that have achieved your desired outcome? (In the purpose of making this exercise simple, I will pretend that the outcome is to be thin and use a thin person as the role model). Where are the thin people? When are they? With whom? What is their environment? For example, you could think of places like the produce department in the grocery store. You can see them in their kitchen cooking healthy food. You can see them at the gym with other people that like to exercise. You can see what clothes they have in their closet. See all the places where the thin people hang out and all their material possessions.

For each square, take the time to see everything you need to see, hear and feel. The same way we have done all the other exercises so far.

Step four: Behaviours

Open your eyes and now step into the next square and pretend it is labelled: Behaviours. As you close your eyes again, ask yourself what do the thin people do in that environment? See everything that would be part of their behaviour. Putting healthy food in their carts at the grocery store, doing squats at the gym, running, eating small portions or whatever comes to your mind when you ask yourself what thin people do. Again, take the time to go through each behaviour or action that you suspect thin people do in those places.

Step five: Skills

The next square is called: Skills. Open your eyes for a second in order to step into it. What are the capabilities that thin people have in order to be able to do these behaviours in these places? What skills do they have? What is required in order to be able to exercise and eat well? Do they have knowledge of healthy food? Are they good at planning meals? Are they good at fitting their workouts in? Are they good at going to bed early? Are they organized?

Step six: Beliefs and values

Open your eyes and step into the next square labelled: Beliefs and Values. What beliefs guide thin people? What do they believe about themselves that allows them to be thin? What is important to thin people? What do they value? Do they value health? Do they believe that their self is set at a thin version of themselves and that, no matter how, their behaviours will always guide them to go back to this set truth about what they are supposed to feel like and look like? Is healthy food important to them? Do they believe that taking the time to pack a lunch is worth the few minutes in the morning? Are they self-confident? Do they believe in themselves?

Step seven: Identity

Again, open and close your eyes for the transition into the next square titled Identity. Who are the thin people? What kind of people are they? In your ideal outcome, what identity do they have? Who are they? Are they genuinely healthy people that shine and radiate happiness?

Step eight: Life purpose

Quickly blink in order to step into the last square: Life Purpose. What is the mission of the thin people? Who else are they serving other than themselves? What vision do they have? Are they able to be a better mother because they don't have to carry all those extra pounds? Are they better to their kids and spouse? Are they able to have a successful career because they have extra time to focus on it as they don't have to spend time worrying about their weight? Are they inspiring others and making their genuine happiness contagious?

Step nine: Backward merge

Now take this life purpose and apply it to yourself. Fully merge the life purpose of the thin people with yours. Make it yours. Integrate it as your new purpose. Take a step back and bring this life purpose into the identity square where you will now fully immerse yourself into the identity of the thin people. You are now a thin person. You are now a genuinely healthy person that shines and radiates happiness. Step back into each square, into beliefs and values, skills, behaviours and environment and apply the responses that you had envisioned to yourself.

Step ten: Fully embody your desired outcome

Step back completely and enjoy an exhilarating moment fully immersed in your desired outcome.

KEY CONCEPTS:

ACT AND MERGE

In order to fully integrate our desired outcome, we have to act as if we had already achieved it and immerse ourselves in each neurological levels to embody each area of ourselves. This process allows to turn the acting into a fully merged reality.

CHAPTER 30

AM I FIXED FOR GOOD NOW?

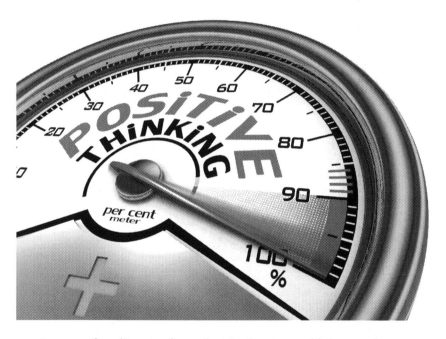

A m I fixed? 50% of people who begin a self-directed program will drop out in the first 6 months. When we are not being monitored, we decrease our chances of success. It is because we lack the mental key.

Is writing your desired well-formed outcome enough? Can you just store it in a drawer now and completely forget about it? Is doing any of these exercises once, all back to back, enough? You must keep re-doing them until they are part of your way of being. Until they become your daily routine. Until you have a natural habit of amplifying and anchoring positive feelings. Until you can easily act a successful behaviour and make it become yours.

Success is the sum of small efforts, repeated day in day out.
Robert Collier

Keep surrounding yourself with positive people. Just like you need to eat every day, you also need to feed your brain every day. In the next few chapters, you will learn how to prevent negative distracting thoughts from interfering. You will be given tools to cope with special circumstances. You will make a plan B and prepare for uncontrollable factors and learn tricks to maintain your new body.

KEY CONCEPTS:

AM I FIXED FOR GOOD?

We need to continue to apply all that we have learned already in our daily lives and prepare a plan for what we can foresee as uncontrollable circumstances.

CHAPTER 31

AWARE

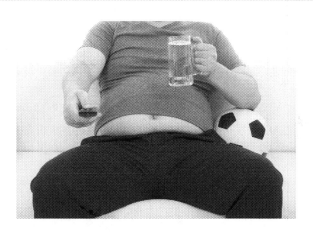

ARE YOU CHOOSING YOUR LIFE?

ware. Did you know that once the average American reaches 60 years old, they have spent about 10 years in front of the television?

Without making any judgment here, I can say that that would be totally fine if it was actually the result of someone's desire to do so. Unfortunately, most of them look back at their lives and say: "I wish I had spent more time with my family, or opened up a business, or called my friends more often, or spent more time on my health and went to the gym, but I had no TIME." And yet, they spent 10 years in front of the T.V.!!

The concept of choice is necessary to understand to be able to be in charge of your life. There are two major aspects to choosing. Firstly, the YES portion of it. A choice is a result of a desire, or not. When you choose something, you say YES to it. The other portion of the choice is the NO portion of it. When you say YES to something, by definition, you say NO to everything else. So whenever you decide to do something, you are putting everything else on the back burner. Make sure to set your priorities and that what you choose is really what you want to do. For some people, their friends and families, their biggest dreams, their health, their sleep, etc. are too often what is left behind while some unimportant matters are chosen to occupy their precious time.

What are you going to say "no" to when you say "yes" to be healthy and slim? If you choose to be healthy, you may need to say "no" to going to the pub on Friday night. Or you may make a positive intention to go to the pub to enjoy seeing your friends, but choose to eat at home first, and then just order something healthy at the pub.

Spend your leisure time wisely. Time is not wasted if you're doing what you want to do. The key word is intention. If you have important priorities to address and make the conscious decision to sit on a bench and do nothing for an hour to clear your mind, it is fine. If you choose to do nothing and you enjoy it, you are spending your time intentionally. If you spend your time intentionally, then it's not wasted and you will have no regrets. The problems occur when we get caught into wasting time un-intentionally.

Sometimes there are things that you do that are not intentional. There are moments of your precious time wasted on things that are not serving you. You need to prepare a plan for what you are going to say "NO" to.

KEY CONCEPTS:

AWARE

We tend to let life pass by without taking charge. It is necessary to understand that saying yes to your new life means saying no to some parts of the old one.

CHAPTER 32

ANTICIPATE

nticipate. Most likely, the reason why you have been unsuccessful in the past is because you did not know that there were other choices and other alternatives to the behaviours that were causing you to fail.

People make the best choices they can at any given time with the resources that are available to them. The more choices you have, the more you become aware of other options, and the more it empowers you and gives you the tools to change.

It is not your personal history that makes you who you are. It is your response to it with the choices that you have available at the time. You can choose what behaviour you want to execute and program them in advance.

We only do the best with what we have. We can never judge anyone. So make sure you avoid judging your past and don't be hard on yourself. In the following exercise, when we go back to an old unwanted behaviour, the only purpose is to identify what triggered this behaviour and replace it with something else more useful. We have the mental skills to see what we don't want and to replace it with what we do want. Change is the only constant in life. Everything in life is temporary. Be in charge of the change that will happen to you, the direction you will go, and what you will become. Don't wait for life to happen to you.

The best way to predict the future is to create it.
Peter F. Drucker

A friend of mine recently purchased one of those wrist devices that calculate your number of daily steps. It even comes with an app on her phone where she can enter the food that she eats and it will help her identify how many calories she has consumed and spent during the day. The calories-in-calories-out technique is something that has worked for her. I personally have one of these watches and I am using it mainly to track my sleep. She did not know that this watch could do that. I taught her how to find that information in the app and we started comparing our sleep patterns. Mine said that I had slept 8 hours and 16 minutes and then it described my sleep quality. I had been awake one time during 8 hours, I had been restless 6 times and I had spent 9 minutes alternating between awake and restless. Her numbers were really different. She had slept for 9 hours 23 minutes. She had been awake 59 times, restless for 4 hours and had spent 3 hours alternating between awake and restless. She was stunned. Now if you are wondering where I am going with this story, here it comes. She said: "I did not know it was possible to sleep through the night like you do. I knew that my sleep was bad but I did not know the extent of it. I thought that it was normal to turn around and take hours before falling asleep and wake up many times during the night."

This was a huge revelation to her. She did not know. Now that the resource had become available to her, she started tracking her sleep and watched her numbers go down. She kept telling me what a big light bulb moment that had been for her. Now she could start having a good night's sleep because she now knew it was possible. She had increased her choices and she was starting to program her brain to sleep profoundly. Now she believed it could be done.

It is time to foresee what can stand between you and your desired outcome. In this chapter, you will develop a plan B. Let's say you had intended to go for a walk every day, but something got in the way of your intention. Anticipate what could happen and have a plan for it.

First, you will identify the threats. Only you can know what has created your past un-successes. After listing what you think could happen, you will prepare some responses that will keep you on track with your new life.

Here are some examples:

You have experienced in the past that the week goes by without you having had time to exercise. If you see that this could happen again in the future, you will now have a workout schedule ready, prepared in advance with some options and you will commit to it. Don't wait until you're tired to do your planning. We don't think or plan well when we're tired.

If you noticed that you were being "weak" (making poor choices) while grocery shopping, you will now always make a grocery list that supports your food plan and you will stick to it.

If your downfall was the fact that you tend to eat out a lot, you will now know what to order in a junk food restaurant. What can you control? What if you go out for dinner? Look up the menu in advance and identify the healthiest thing on the menu and visualize yourself ordering it. If your co-workers are going for lunch at Dairy Queen, you can go too and have a plan to eat a salad there.

Have a "What if" plan. What if you get called into a meeting at lunch time? You will have a protein shake in your desk that you can quickly mix with water and drink quickly before your meeting.

What if everyone orders dessert? You will ask your friend to order an extra fork and ask for one bite of hers. Or, when it's time to order desert, get up and go to the ladies room. When you come back to the table, it will be too late to order.

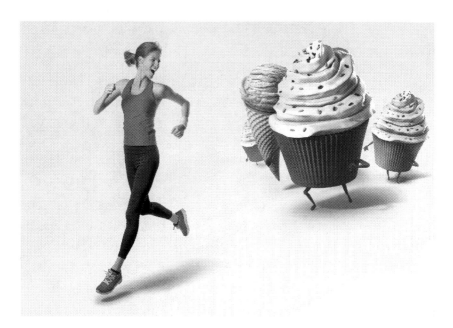

What if you get home too late and you miss your fitness class? Go for a walk instead. Always take control and have a backup plan. What if you feel too tired to exercise? What if you are supposed to workout and you are spent? Prepare a "lazy-workout" for that in advance. What if you feel sick? What can you do instead? Go for a walk instead of a run. You can still do something. If you were going to go for a run and it's raining, what do you do? Grab a hat, and run in the rain.

Maybe one of your friends makes you cookies all the time. Ask her to do you a favour and help support your new lifestyle by giving her baked goods to someone else.

If you eat chocolate when you didn't intend to, forget about it and go home and feed yourself well. Don't feel bad; it's too late for that. Instead, do something positive like clean out the pantry and throw out your junk food.

Set yourself up for success. Don't let yourself be surprised. Know in advance. I know you already have a lot of ideas in your head! You know what distractions present themselves to you! No more surprises! Be in charge now. Take control and do a conscious vision and plan for if you don't feel you're 100%. And always give the 100% you have. Prepare, prepare, prepare. Always have a plan B. Always prepare for things you can't control.

Obstacles are those frightful things you see when you take your eyes off your goal.

Henry Ford

Here you go. List some obstructions that could get in the way of your weight loss intentions.

Obstructions

- Anticipate the things that could get in the way

    1. _____

    2. _____

    3. _____

    4. _____

    5. _____

    6. _____

    7. _____

    8. _____

    9. _____

    10. _____

- Find an alternative for them – what's your plan B?

1. _____

2. _____

3. _____

4. _____

5. _____

6. _____

7. _____

8. _____

9. _____

10. _____

KEY CONCEPTS:

ANTICIPATE

You more than likely know some scenarios that could get in the way of your new lifestyle.

By anticipating these situations, you can plan ahead what you will choose to do instead.

CHAPTER 33

ALTERNATE BEHAVIOUR

Alternate behaviour. Now that we have taken care of anticipating what could happen, it is now time to install the alternate behaviours. This chapter will show you a technique in order to allow you to choose and install an alternate behaviour in case of a threat to your desired outcome.

This technique is similar to the *New You* and the *Neutralize the Past* techniques that we saw in chapters 24 and 25. We identified a negative feeling, emotion or behaviour that we wanted to change and we replaced it with something else. The Alternate Behaviour technique will allow you to identify an unwanted behaviour that could occur in your journey to achieving your positive outcome - remember the desires that you elicited in the DESIRE section of the book? - and we will install positive responses instead. It is like planning ahead what you will need to do differently. You will replace your past weight-loss unsuccessful behaviours by new ones that will serve you better.

Step one: Identify the behaviour to choose an alternative for

Think of an obstacle that could get in the way and how you used to react in the past. Now, with your desired outcome in mind, elicit a behaviour that you would like to do instead. For example, you used to have a hard time resisting a piece of cake at a birthday party or you used to get the munchies at night while watching television. Pick a specific problem and do the full Alternate Behaviour technique for each problem that could potentially occur.

Step two: Find the trigger

Go back to a moment where you had a negative response and identify what was the exact trigger for it. There was a moment where a specific stimulus caused you to generate the unwanted behaviour. With the example of the cake at a birthday party, is it when the cake comes to the table that you decide that you will have a piece? Is it when it is sliced and handed to you on a plate? For the example of the munchies at night-time, it could be when there is a commercial that you think about getting up and going to get something to eat or it could be before you even sit down, already planning a snack for your television watching session.

Step three: Choose your ideal response

As you think about the trigger, think about what other behaviour you would like to install in your unconscious mind instead. For the cake example, it could be to see yourself saying: "No, thank you, I am full" as you are having a genuine impression of feeling full and honestly feel completely indifferent to the cake. For the television munchies example, it could be seeing yourself boiling some water to make to some herbal tea and seeing yourself enjoy it as you watch your favourite show.

Step four: Install the alternate the behaviour

Get the old picture of the unwanted behaviour in your head. Associate yourself in the image, meaning that you are seeing it through your own eyes. Make the picture big and bright and add lots of detail.

Now, make an image of the alternate behaviour in a dissociated way, meaning that you are looking at yourself doing the new behaviour. Take this picture and make it very small (coin-sized) and place it in the corner of your vision.

Take this coin-sized picture of the new behaviour and make it go away, further and further, as if you wanted to send it out to the universe, all the way out to the moon, as if it was being stretched out far away on a giant sling shot. When you are ready, launch this new behaviour image as a rocket towards you. As you see the image getting bigger and richer and bolder, moving rapidly towards you, send the old image in the opposite direction, in its own sling shot. Make the old picture darker and smaller and less powerful as it is flying away from you.

Exhale loudly as the two images pass beside each other, as the old behaviour leaves completely to make room solely for the new behaviour. As the new image hits you, associate through it, meaning, start seeing the action as if from your own eyes. As opposed to looking at yourself drinking a cup of tea, you are now seeing the cup of tea in your own hands and the living room and the television in front of you.

Step five: Amplify the new behaviour.

Make the picture bigger and brighter. Make it bold and beautiful. Feel an amazing feeling rush through you - you can use your anchored positive feeling here - and tell yourself that this is the way you will behave from now on.

Step six: Repeat.

Now remember that your unconscious mind likes repetition. You will quickly go from one image to the other and repeat the process at least ten times. Exhale loudly each time the slingshots launch the images to alternate them. I cannot stress enough the importance of doing this repetitively and quickly.

Step seven: Test.

Now verify that you have done the process correctly. Think of the trigger moment. Feel that someone is offering you a piece of birthday cake on a plate. Go there now as if it was really happening. What behaviour comes to mind? The first thing that comes out should be the "No thank you" behaviour.

The idea is to add choices and resources. When you take away choices, other compensating behaviours can occur. If you want to make better choices, decide what you would like instead. The more you have pre-planned your alternate behaviours, the easier it is to go through your daily life that will lead to a thinner version of yourself. Find the tools you need and have them available. Buy yourself a vegetable tray and a fruit tray each week and you will eat them because they're already prepared and they're in your fridge. Hard boil 5 eggs for yourself this week and put them in the fridge so you can grab one every day on your way to work. Sign up for a fitness class and always have your workout clothes and shoes ready in a bag in your car. Make it easy for yourself. Have resources available. As you surf through your week, you will use these resources.

KEY CONCEPTS:

ALTERNATE BEHAVIOUR

You can switch an unwanted behaviour to a more serving one by creating two specific images and using a sling-shot-technique to exchange one image with the other.

CHAPTER 34

ACCOUNTABLE

Accountable. This chapter will help you commit to some actions. You can't reach your new lifestyle if you think that *someday* you will start eating well and *someday* you will start exercising. *Someday* is a code for "never". Your someday has yet to come and will forever be this unnamed day. Turn someday into TODAY. You can be as healthy as you want to be. Now.

In order to be accountable to yourself, make a list of concrete actions or behaviours that you will commit to doing. Choose your actions according to the areas that you identified in chapter 12 DEDICATE and DIVIDE. Remember when you filled out your wheel?

List three things that you are going to do this week if you want to bring your pie slices up closer to 10. We are not aiming for a 10 necessarily. Just aim for one more point. If you have given yourself a 4, what can cause this 4 to increase to a 5?

Choose 1 slice of your wheel first. Baby steps, remember? Write one to three things that you can do today in order to increase the number by 1.

I choose to work on the slice called:

_____

List 3 things you will do this Week to make this slice of the pie go up of one point: **short term action**

1. _____

2. _____

3. _____

Remember that these commitments can be anchored, amplified, installed with the alternate behaviour technique and everything you have learned. Take these actions and actualize them with the tools that have worked for you so far.

Once the actions you committed to above are easy and on-going new habits, you will work on the following three new things: **long term actions**

1. _____

2. _____

3. _____

There is power in setting up the intentions and installing them into your unconscious mind. Now that you know how this works, you will constantly be amazed at how much your life has shifted and changed in light of all this new knowledge.

KEY CONCEPTS:

ACCOUNTABLE

By writing down the specific and concrete actions you want to commit to, you are making yourself accountable.

You want to use all the tools you have learned so far to process these new commitments in your brain.

CHAPTER 35

AUTHENTIC

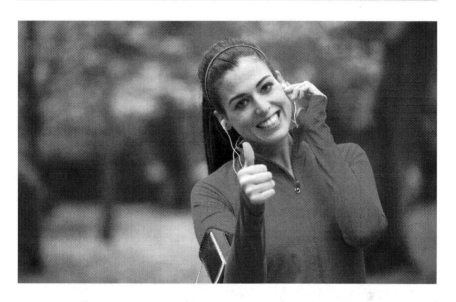

A uthentic. Now that you are mastering the art of programming your brain, and are fully excited and motivated, you may wonder how to keep this going. How can you feel fully, genuinely authentic?

My mom used to tell me that we need to eat food everyday to feed our body but we also need to feed our brain daily. I have developed the habit of downloading audio books that I listen to in the morning as I get ready for my day. Jack Canfield once said: "You can't put your hand in a bucket of glue, without some of that glue sticking to your hand." So I like to "audio-read" biographies of successful people, their stories, how they did it and what lessons I can learn from them. I find that audiobooks work well for me as they can play in the background in the kitchen when I cook or in my car while I drive. It is all food for the soul.

Here are some of my favourite books:

- A New Earth by Eckhart Tolle
- Awaken the Giant Within by Anthony Robbins
- Change your Brain, change your Body by Daniel G. Amen
- Gateway to Success and Hapiness by Og Mandino
- Get the Life you Want by Richard Bendler
- Good to Great by Jim Collins
- Great by Choice by Jim Collins
- Happy for no Reason by Marci Shimoff
- How to Create the Life you Want by Wayne Dwyer
- How to Overcome your self limiting beliefs & achieve anything you want by Omar Johnson
- Le Millionnaire by Marc Fisher
- Mindset by Carol S. Dweck
- Power vs Force by David R. Hawkins
- Road to Valor by Aili and Andres McConnon
- Take a shot by Dave Morrow and Jake Steinfeld
- The 7 Habits of Highly Effective People by Stephen R. Covey
- The 8th Habit by Stephen R. Covey
- The Art of Thinking Clearly by Rolf Dobelli
- The Diet Fix by Yoni Freedhoff
- The foundation of Succesful Change by Zig Ziglar
- The Greatest salesman in the world by Og Mandino
- The Life-changing magic of tidying up by Marie Kondo
- The Motivation Manifesto by Brendon Burchard
- The Purple Cow by Seth Godin
- The Rise of Superman by Steven Kotler
- The Ultimate Gift by Jim Stovall
- The Ultimate Introduction to NLP by Richard Bandler
- The Untethered Soul by Michael A. Singer
- Way of the Peaceful Warrior by Dan Millman
- Who moved my cheese by Spencer Johnson
- Why People Fail by Siimon Reynolds

Start your day off by listening to positive, motivating audiotapes on your iPod or iPhone. If we don't motivate ourselves, then who will? Stay focused. If it's too hard for you to stay motivated, hire a coach. Or join a class with a group of friends who will help you stay on track and stay motivated. Timing is important. If right now for example, you're going through a divorce, you're quitting smoking, changing jobs etc. then right now is probably not the best time for you to start this weight loss journey. Remember to do one thing at a time, take baby steps.

What are you going to do to stay motivated? It's easy after you've just been fed positive information and tools. Your homework now is to put in place the tools you will need to stay motivated. Getting into a good state is mandatory when we are learning and implementing new good habits. If you take problems too seriously, you make them more real. Eating sweets is not a personality trait; it is just a bad habit. Building good feelings should be something you do every day.

- What are you going to do to stay motivated?

    1. _____

    2. _____

    3. _____

Exchange phone numbers with people who motivate you. Hire a personal trainer or a coach that will hold you accountable for the actions you've committed to. Do some reading and research. Download audio books. Tell the whole world about how motivated you are about your new life. Choose to spend less time with negative people. Start on this journey with a friend. Give this book to everyone you know so that you are all on the same page. Use whatever works. Implement some tools to keep you motivated and make them work for you.

KEY CONCEPTS:

AUTHENTIC

By committing to feeding your brain with positive information on a regular basis, you increase your daily level of motivation.

Chose some techniques you will use to stay motivated.

CHAPTER 36

ADOPT THE TOOTHPASTE PHILOSOPHY

Adopt the toothpaste philosophy. I spent a short time in Thailand. At the end of trip through the main cities, I was fortunate to visit a small island where we met a young boy working on the beach, bringing us fresh coconut water every day. I was stunned by the way people lived in Thailand. This country was a happy organized chaos. Just in Bangkok, where millions of people try to get their spot on the road, and where the traffic alone is enough to give us North Americans a heart attack, the people seem to be genuinely happy. They smile. They are patient. They give way to each other with a friendly gesture (unlike the frequent road rage and fingers that we can witness on our roads here). So I asked our new friend on the beach how I could learn from him about this wonderful way of living. He told me about a philosophy that he had been living by all his life. I named it the toothpaste philosophy.

He said that in life, we all have challenges and we all have about 800 decisions to make every day; the same philosophy needs to be applied to all of them. In the morning, when your alarm goes off, you have to decide if you will get up right away or if you will choose to snooze for an extra 9 minutes. If your favourite shirt is in the laundry basket, you will have to choose another one to wear. If you are having a bad hair day, you may choose to wear a pony tail instead. If you run out of toothpaste, you may need to squeeze the tube to get a little drop in order to brush your teeth. Your day goes on and you might even almost get run over by a car on your way to work. You might get there only to find out that the doors of the store you work at are closed indefinitely and you are now out of a job. Perhaps your best friend calls you to announce that she is going through a divorce with her husband. You might stop at the hospital where your father has been for the past few weeks, only to find out that he has lung cancer and doesn't have much longer to live. Perhaps you get back to your car and find a parking ticket on the windshield. On your way home, you might stop at the drugstore, remembering somehow that you needed toothpaste.

Hopefully, all these events would not happen to you in a single day. But following my Thai friend's philosophy, all these events can be addressed with the same type of response and the same attitude. Our reaction to the events happening throughout the day needs to be the same as the response we gave when we ran out of toothpaste. You squeezed the tube and thought to yourself: "Well, I will just go and get another tube later on today on my way home." This was the way my beach boy lived his life. He perceived every challenge as if it was just another one of the 800 things that would be happening to him that day. He never let things affect his mood and he accepted the facts, understanding that the external events are only there to build who we are and that the rollercoaster of emotions that we are putting ourselves through every day is not worth the stress we are putting on our body.

I admit that the example above is exaggerated and it's natural that emotions get in the way of our judgement sometimes. Of course, we would react to a terrible tragedy that may have occurred. But sometimes we allow ourselves to get all cranked up at the seat belt in our car for not complying with our wishes or the way we react when someone interrupts what we are doing. We would get more joy out of life if we adopted the toothpaste philosophy and reacted to most events of our day as "no big deal". Studies show that the big dramas in life like the loss of a loved one or a job, divorce, etc. are not the events that cause the damaging stress. Because usually, we take the means that we need to face these big challenges and get tools to overcome them. We usually also get support and most of all, we accept the support from others in these situations. The damaging stress mostly comes from the little things in life that we get so upset about and that don't really matter at all at the end of the day.

I read an anonymous sign the other day that said: "I still have trouble in life, but it is not a problem anymore". It is just about the way we react to the external pressure.

KEY CONCEPTS:

ADOPT THE TOOTHPASTE PHILOSOPHY

Take the drama out of your life by adopting the toothpaste philosophy. When something goes wrong, pretend that it is as impact free and temporary as running out of toothpaste. Just go buy another tube.

CHAPTER 37

APPRECIATE

Appreciate. Take the time to enjoy life and your successes. Use the D.N.A. System for everything you would like to change in your life. Weight loss is only one issue where this amazing system has been successful.

Now you know the system. First, you start with setting up your DESIRE and use the tools that I have provided you to decide on a compelling outcome. Then, you clean up your past in order to create a NEW YOU, free of negative emotions and limiting beliefs. And lastly, you ACTUALIZE your desire with the programming techniques that you have learned and make sure your NEW YOU is permanent.

As you create your new life, take some time to slow down and appreciate little things. Train yourself to feel good, like you train your muscles. Feeling good is a physiological response so you can train it. Be excited and enthusiastic! Whatever life brings you, you are now in control of how you can respond to it. Chose to respond in a dynamic and fun way. You are making it up anyways! You might as well create your new life expecting it to be absolutely amazing!

Why wait to feel good when you can now choose when you want to feel good. On demand. Why wait for something great to happen in order for us to feel good? Because when you decide to feel good who is going to make you feel good? Who will generate the feeling good emotions for you? You will! So why wait? Feel great now! You know how many times we say: "Someday, we will look back at this and laugh about it". Why wait? Might as well laugh now and get it over with right away! Have you ever heard yourself say: "I will be happy when this week is over"? Why wait for the week to be over to be happy. Just be happy now.

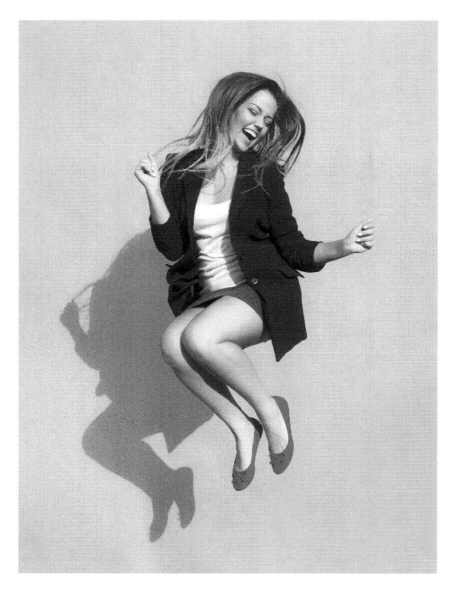

Remember that you have the ability to manage your state. Make sure you choose your life and who you surround yourself with.

Create a world where it is easy to dream what you want to be, write down what you want and do what you wrote. And remember to always do one thing at a time, consistently.

Don't just Be. Be Your Best.

KEY CONCEPTS:

APPRECIATE

Enjoy your life. You only live once.

CHAPTER 38

ABOUT THE AUTHOR - WHO IS NATHALIE PLAMONDON-THOMAS?

About me. I am an award winning fitness professional, an NLP Master Practitioner and Life Coach. I was born in a small town in Quebec, Canada. You know how a lot of people have that kind of story that they suffered in their childhood or had a rough go at something in their life and then they turned their life around, learned from the events and then became stronger? Well, that could not be further away from the truth for me.

I was raised by highly intelligent and spiritually advanced parents, in a positive and loving environment. My parents were really into motivation and positive thinking. And to this day, they are still the most supportive and caring people on the planet. They are my coaches, my friends, my counsellors, my fan club and I really look up to them. They wired me to be the person that I am today at a very young age.

In my childhood, they didn't put a gate by the stairs when my brother and I were babies because they never wanted to imply that we could fall. They would instead say: "Be careful around there". They didn't say: "Don't fall" or "Get out of there or you will fall". If they needed me to bring a full glass of water to the table they would just say: "use a strong steady hand and bring this glass successfully to the table" instead of saying: "don't spill it!", creating anxiety around the action of carrying the water. Can you see the nuance?

There were signs everywhere in the house with motivational phrases like: "You can be everything you want"; "Yes you can"; "You will miss 100% of the shots you won't take"; "If you're going to do it, do it right"; "There is no luck, you deserve everything you get"; and "Luck is a word that was created by people who are too lazy to do what they have to do". My father's favourite saying was: "NOT ABLE TO is dead, his little sister's name is: TRY."

On Sundays, we were not going to church (although we are Christian Catholics), but instead, my parents would make us sit in the living room to listen to some motivational tape cassettes from Jean-Marc Chaput, Zig Ziglar, Og Mandino, etc. So, needless to say, I was introduced to positive thinking at a very young age.

I lived in Quebec for a big chunk of my life. I then moved to Toronto, Ontario in my twenties, where I studied Neuro-Linguistic Programming (NLP) and Life Coaching. I now live in White Rock, British Columbia and recently completed my Master Practitioner Certification with the Robinson Group.

The name of my company is DNA Life Coaching. I do believe that everybody has whatever they need inside their DNA in order to obtain, achieve and be whatever they put their mind to. More than a company mission statement, I believe that my life purpose is to motivate and inspire others to be their best.

I got my first "calling" to help people at a very young age. My parents would not read us Disney stories at night. They would either sing us a song to put us to sleep with their guitar (which explains my love for music), or they would tell us motivational stories. Here is my favourite bedtime story: It is about an old man on the beach, who was throwing back the starfishes in the sea, one by one. A little girl asked him: "What are you doing sir?" and the old man responded: "I am saving the starfishes from dying, as the tide brought them to shore, they will dry and die if I don't throw them back in the sea." The little girl looked at the endlessly long beach and said: "But sir, no offence, but there are so many, you can't save them all! It doesn't really make a difference." And the old man responded, as he was showing the little girl that starfish that he was holding in his hands: "Well my dear, for this particular starfish, it makes a whole world of difference." I was thinking: "When I grow up, I will be a starfish saviour and save them all, one at a time!" And the rest is history.

If you can't feed a hundred people, then feed just one.
Mother Teresa

So now, I work with clients one-on-one and I help people be what they want to be. I have also been teaching fitness classes and personal training for over 27 years, and I am a Nutrition and Wellness Specialist. Fitness and Nutrition have always been my favourite platform in order to help people be their best. I also work with kids in schools, which gives me even wider audience to impact and improve people's lives because I believe if certain values are planted at a young age, they have a better chance to find their roots and flourish.

I was blessed to be given the tools to constantly boost my self-confidence so that I can go about living a life where I believe that I can do anything and succeed at everything I touch. My mother used to tell me all the time: "You are great at everything you do". Even today, there isn't a day when I don't hear my mother's voice saying it to me over and over.

A funny example of how deep the roots of this belief have been planted inside me is to tell you how I choose to react to certain situations in life. I do a lot of seminars and speaking engagements. Sometimes, in my seminars, I see some people with their arms crossed. Most strategists would tell you that it means that they are not liking what they are hearing. Instead, I choose to believe that they are cold. It is a much simpler version which serves me much better at being at my best and continue to use all my skills in order to create rapport with my audience. By not letting this influence me in a negative way, I remain at my best and soon enough, I get them to "warm-up" to me. If I chose to belief that it is because I am not interesting, I may lose my self-confidence and my whole seminar might be put in jeopardy. It's the same if someone rolls their eyes, I tell myself that what I just said contradicts something that they had heard before and what I am saying makes so much more sense and they are rolling their eyes at the old information that they used to believe. I don't really know what they are thinking. I cannot mind-read. So I am making up a story anyways. I might as well make up a story that serves me. I am sure that if one day someone tells me to go to hell, I will think it is a new restaurant downtown!

THANK YOU

Thank you to the following people who inspired me and/or contributed to this book:

My parents Micheline and Yves Plamondon for their constant inspiration and support, Pam Rigden from Fitness Unlimited who introduced me to NLP 8 years ago, Lynn Robinson from the Robinson Group, an amazing Master Trainer and friend with whom I completed my Master in NLP, Suzanne Doyle-Ingram from SDI Communications, Jennifer Baynton, Stacy Thomas and of course my husband Duff Thomas for his continuous support.

Printed in the United States
By Bookmasters